Humanising Psych Mental Health Care

T0227395

The challenge of the person-centred approach

Rachel Freeth

Psychiatrist in General Adult Psychiatry
Gloucestershire

Forewords by

Brian Thorne

Emeritus Professor of Counselling

and

Mike Shooter

Consultant Psychiatrist
Immediate Past President, Royal College of Psychiatrists

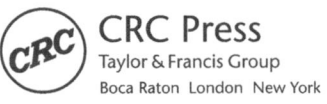

CRC Press
Taylor & Francis Group
Boca Raton London New York

CRC Press is an imprint of the
Taylor & Francis Group, an **informa** business

CRC Press
Taylor & Francis Group
6000 Broken Sound Parkway NW, Suite 300
Boca Raton, FL 33487-2742

© 2007 Rachel Freeth
CRC Press is an imprint of Taylor & Francis Group, an Informa business

No claim to original U.S. Government works

International Standard Book Number-13: 978-1-85775-619-7 (Hardback)

This book contains information obtained from authentic and highly regarded sources. Reasonable efforts have been made to publish reliable data and information, but the author and publisher cannot assume responsibility for the validity of all materials or the consequences of their use. The authors and publishers have attempted to trace the copyright holders of all material reproduced in this publication and apologize to copyright holders if permission to publish in this form has not been obtained. If any copyright material has not been acknowledged please write and let us know so we may rectify in any future reprint.

Except as permitted under U.S. Copyright Law, no part of this book may be reprinted, reproduced, transmitted, or utilized in any form by any electronic, mechanical, or other means, now known or hereafter invented, including photocopying, microfilming, and recording, or in any information storage or retrieval system, without written permission from the publishers.

For permission to photocopy or use material electronically from this work, please access www.copyright.com (http://www.copyright.com/) or contact the Copyright Clearance Center, Inc. (CCC), 222 Rosewood Drive, Danvers, MA 01923, 978-750-8400. CCC is a not-for-profit organization that provides licenses and registration for a variety of users. For organizations that have been granted a photocopy license by the CCC, a separate system of payment has been arranged.

Trademark Notice: Product or corporate names may be trademarks or registered trademarks, and are used only for identification and explanation without intent to infringe.

Visit the Taylor & Francis Web site at
http://www.taylorandfrancis.com

and the CRC Press Web site at
http://www.crcpress.com

Contents

Foreword

As someone who has devoted most of his professional life to the practice of person-centred therapy and the advancement of the person-centred approach, I find Dr Rachel Freeth's courageous book serves as a striking commentary on much that has characterised my own experience over the years. Like her, I have known the disenchantment and the mounting anger engendered by the emergence of a culture permeated by rampant consumerism and the obsession with so-called cost-effectiveness allied to a profound distrust in the human spirit. I, too, have struggled to retain a sense of personal integrity in the face of bureaucratic processes and managerial strategies induced by a mentality with the apparent intent of subjecting everyone to scarcely veiled surveillance in order to make the subsequent attribution of blame the more clear-cut. Unlike Rachel, however, I have also known a different era. Nor have I had the misfortune to work as a psychiatrist in today's National Health Service, which, as far as its response to mental distress is concerned, seems to become progressively more dysfunctional. At her age, I had the good fortune to be the founding Director of a university counselling service committed to the person-centred approach and inspired by the work of Carl Rogers, who was still very much alive and power-fully influential. Those were the days – in the mid 1970s – when it still seemed possible that the idealism and the belief in human creativity which had char-acterised the previous decade might ultimately triumph and the world of education become the crucible in which the seeds of such transformation could be sown and nurtured. As I have read Rachel's book it has been immensely reassuring to discover that, despite deepening pessimism over the years, my fundamental hope has not diminished. I have learned, however, that hope is not to be confused with optimism. It is rather the antidote to despair and, as such, it can face the worst and not be overcome. Such hope also knows something of what the theologian, W. H. Vanstone, once called the stature of waiting.

When Rachel, already a psychiatrist, came to the University of East Anglia in the 1990s to train as a person-centred therapist, the agonising tensions that run throughout this book were already manifest. It was clear that she had known profound suffering both in her own life and in the lives of her patients but she was also full of an apparently irrational hope. Like many others who present themselves for training in the person-centred approach she had found in the writings of Carl Rogers a confirmation of what she had always somehow known but had never been able fully to articulate. She discovered that, like her, he had a deep trust in the ability of human beings to flourish if they are offered a relationship in which they experience unqualified acceptance, deep under-standing and the respect due to someone of infinite value. Not that the offering of such a relationship is a simple matter for it demands of the one who offers, be it therapist or friend, a level of skill, commitment and self-acceptance which is increasingly rare in our competitive, acquisitive and fearful culture. During her training, however, Rachel discovered not only that such relationships are possible but also that they work. When she returned to psychiatry, what she had always instinctively known was now firmly buttressed by an elegant theory and proven practice.

In many ways this book is the story of what it has meant for the psychiatrist/ person-centred counsellor to remain hopeful and resilient in the face of the ever-deepening crisis that she has experienced in the powerfully drug-orientated and medicalised world of NHS psychiatry. Much of what she relates is deeply shocking for it points to an environment where the humanity of doctors, nurses and patients alike is constantly endangered by a prevailing alienation where the dignity of persons is lost in the frantic attempt to keep chaos at bay by refusing relationship in the interests of symptom control and the containment of emotional expression. We learn of exhausted and demoralised doctors who themselves tremble on the verge of breakdown and long for part-time employment or early retirement as they attempt to respond to impossible caseloads within the context of insane policies. Not that the person-centred therapeutic community escapes all criticism. Person-centred practitioners are taken to task for their often ignorant or contemptuous attitude towards psychiatry and their failure to acknowledge both the dedicated commitment and expert knowledge of many psychiatrists and the intractable difficulties of the system in which most are compelled to operate. It is at this interface that Rachel Freeth, thanks to her two disciplines, embodies a hope and a vision which can vanquish despair. As she seeks to be the interpreter between two worlds, we glimpse a future where psychiatrists and person-centred therapists will collaborate in the healing of persons in the context of a culture which has drawn back at the eleventh hour from the brink of self-destruction. The day where the sanctity of persons and the creation of community become the hallmarks of a civilised society may be far distant but it is books like this which keep the vision alive and serve as beacons in the current darkness.

Brian Thorne
Norwich
January 2007

Foreword

'To travel hopefully is a better thing than to arrive, and the success is to labour.'
(Robert Louis Stevenson. *Virginibus Puerisque*. 'El Dorado')

You would think that writing a foreword would be a relatively easy task. You read the book or, more often one suspects, you skim through it. You dash off a few paragraphs of fulsome praise or pad out the contents page. You are careful to advertise your own achievements in the field. You include it in your cv as if you had written the book itself. And you sit back and wait for the acknowledgement. So why did I find writing this foreword a much less comfortable experience?

To begin with, Rachel is an excoriatingly honest writer. To produce a textbook about patients, their assessment, diagnosis and treatment might be laborious, even physically exhausting, but rarely an emotional challenge. Person-centred therapy cannot be reduced to such objectivity; it begins and ends with the self. To write about it, just as in its practice, the author must examine her own life. Rachel does so in a way that is both brave and unsettling.

More than this, to pay her proper credit the book demands the reader examine his own life in return. In my case, it arrived as I approached retirement. An end, as I thought, to clinical work in the NHS and in the administration of my College. It forced me to look back at what had brought me into the job in the first place and what had kept me there for a quarter of a century of doubts and disillusionment. It made me realise that what I had been searching for through all my career changes, from lawyer, to newspaper reporter, to teacher, and finally to doctor, was the wisdom that lies at the core of Rachel's book. A face-to-face relationship of humanity, humility and honesty that has all but disappeared from modern medicine.

It made me think of my own periods of depression, of a therapist who valued me for what I was, rather than what so many people wanted me to be, at a time when I loathed myself and imagined that everyone must do likewise. It made me aware that it was this sensitivity that had carried me into psychiatry in due course. It made me feel lucky that I had trained in a hospital run as a therapeutic community in which people like Carl Rogers were gurus whose principles we clung to like a mantra. But above all, it challenged me about whether I had maintained those principles as firmly as Rachel has done in her own practice.

For the true person-centred approach, as opposed to the lip-service paid to it in statements of government policy, is not easy to implement. It is difficult to measure against the randomised controlled trial of medication and other organic treatments. It cannot achieve the superficial, short-term, CORE-scored results of cognitive behavioural therapy. It relies on the narrative evidence of what life feels like to the individual patient rather than what that general category of patient must feel because the science says so. And it has a battle to establish its worth in the competitive world of commissioning, where success is judged on through-put of patients not the quality of their lives.

How scary all this can be! Trusting in the patient's 'actualising tendency' means taking risks in a risk-aversive climate where guidelines are laid down for everything, therapists may be punished by the CMC for not keeping the faith and patients punished for their resistance by legal, physical and medicinal incarceration. We are asked to treat with unconditional regard those patients who may irritate, frighten or appal us by their behaviour and to empathise with those whose chronic disorder denies us the satisfaction of cure. It may cause us to confront all those unresolved issues in our own lives whose pain we have suppressed in the guise of helping others.

Small wonder that in the face of such challenges we have witnessed what a colleague has called 'the endless retreat from patients'. Some of us go into academic research, some into service management. Some of us climb the structures of our profession, some the slippery slope of NHS politics. All of us are tempted to keep the dangers of patient relationships at a white-coated, technological distance. Rachel has not done so. She has championed the person-centred approach at enormous cost to herself and is able to write about it without the merest trace of hypocrisy.

This is not a book for the faint-hearted. There is no easy framework here to aid your understanding of the medical world and your role in it. The book offers no theoretical asylum from the sneers of those who criticise the person-centred approach for its lack of objectivity. It is a tough philosophy, confident in its assertion of subjective principles and everything that flows from them. It provides no guarantee of success and no insurance against failure. But it is more inspiring than anything I have read for a very long time.

Rachel's work has made me realise, like Stevenson, that it is not the comfort of arrival that we should aspire to but the labour of honest travel, being true to our patients and our own beliefs, no matter what difficulties may be thrown in the path. She has made me want to get moving again, to hope for the best but, in the words of another of my favourite authors, if things do not work out, to 'Try again. Fail again. Fail better' (Samuel Beckett. *Worstward Ho*). We should ask no less of ourselves than we do of our patients.

Mike Shooter
January 2007

What is needed, if we are serious about helping people, is to raise this experience called "relationship" to our conscious and careful consideration in order to be able to use it in competent and responsible ways in the best interests of those we serve.

Helen Harris Perlman

... as long as I know how to love I know I'll stay alive ...

'I Will Survive' song lyrics
Gloria Gaynor

For Mum and Dad –
Who loved me enough
To allow me to
Shape my own life.

Acknowledgements

It is a real pleasure to acknowledge the many people whose encouragement and enthusiasm for this project has sustained me during numerous difficult times, and who have given me sufficient inner belief and confidence to embark on it in the first place. I would like to acknowledge in particular Brian Thorne, to whom I am also grateful for providing one of the Forewords for this book. Maggie Pettifer at Radcliffe Publishing also deserves special mention and gratitude for placing faith and trust in me as a writer and who, in a person-centred way, gave me the space, time and understanding I needed to enable the book to evolve naturally. This book has also benefited from the willingness of several people to read drafts of chapters and to provide comment and suggestions. Included here are Richard Bryant-Jefferies, Phill Morgan-Henshaw, Julie Mordin, Catherine Clarke, Paul Evans and Ilse Ferwerda. I would also like to thank Mike Shooter, not only for providing me with the other Foreword, but for the particular brand of caring and humanity he has brought to the psychiatric profession. Finally, I thank my partner Ilse for, amongst other things, tolerating all the times when I am only half listening.

Introduction

'Before you begin a thing, remind yourself that difficulties and delays quite impossible to foresee are ahead. ... You can only see one thing clearly and that is your goal. Form a mental vision of that and cling to it through thick and thin.'

(Kathleen Norris, American Writer, 1880–1966)

Carl Rogers (1902–1987) is a figure not normally associated with contemporary psychiatry. Neither is the person-centred approach that developed from his thinking and practice and those of his co-workers. This is not surprising. In many ways the person-centred approach is the antithesis of current mental health practice that is often, in my view, oppressive and dehumanised. Patients are increasingly 'processed' through a fragmented and mechanistically structured mental health service and the mental health culture regularly demonstrates a failure to recognise the vital importance of relationship with patients as a powerful and necessary healing ingredient. As well as challenging traditional power structures and placing relationship at the centre of the helping endeavour, the person-centred approach presents a positive philosophy of human beings and their growth and recovery potential. It also presents a radical and desperately needed challenge to the culture of medicalisation and exclusive reliance on the medical model.

The aims

In this book I explore the philosophy, theory and practice of the person-centred approach (not to be confused with the sound-bite 'person-centred' as used by politicians and managers) in the context of both contemporary psychiatry and mental health services provided by the UK's National Health Service (NHS). In so doing, I pay attention both to how the person-centred approach can challenge psychiatry and to how mental health services and the NHS present challenges and tensions to person-centred practitioners working in them. I believe that such challenges need to be highlighted and understood for there to be any hope of placing the person-centred approach more on the map within psychiatry and mental health settings. Why the person-centred approach should be on the map in the first place will be argued throughout this book, although whether I argue my case sufficiently to convince a sceptic remains to be seen.

I realise I am ambitious in having for this book four broad aims. First, I want to introduce the person-centred approach and the theory and philosophy of Carl Rogers to mental health professionals and to plug a major gap within the current mental health literature. I believe it is necessary not only to increase the understanding of this approach beyond its more usual association as simply a type of listening, but also to attempt to correct the many misunderstandings that abound. Some of these include the belief that the approach is a form of counselling only suitable for the 'worried well' and that it lacks a comprehensive theory which, at the same time, is seen as a naïve view of human beings. Unfair caricatures of person-centred counsellors depict them to be sentimental, 'touchy-feely' types, who do little more than smile benignly at the client, or who are experts at 'reflecting' what the client has just said.

Whilst mental health nurses used to receive a thorough grounding in the person-centred approach in their training, current training introduces Rogers and the approach in little more than superficial terms. It is often reduced to a set of listening skills rather than presented as a philosophy towards human beings and helping them. As a psychiatrist in training I could easily have progressed in my career with next to no knowledge of the person-centred approach. Furthermore, person-centred therapy is hardly ever offered, if at all, as an approach in which psychiatric trainees can gain some experience of practising psychotherapy. The lowly status of person-centred therapy within psychiatry is also reflected in the fact that it is rarely available as a form of therapy provided by psychological therapy services within secondary care. The person-centred approach is more likely to be encountered as a counselling approach within primary care. Why the person-centred approach is so marginalised and dismissed within mental health services will be apparent throughout this book. Suffice it to say, though, it represents a paradigm that is not for the faint-hearted to practise from, not least because it clashes with the prevailing biomedical paradigm within psychiatry.

Second, as much as mental health professionals could benefit from learning more about the person-centred approach, many person-centred practitioners could benefit from furthering their understanding of the theories and practices of psychiatry and how NHS mental health services function. Psychiatry is often stigmatised through ignorance and misunderstanding and mental health professionals are also caricatured. There is valuable debate to be had between psychiatry and the person-centred approach, but traditional antagonisms need first to be dissolved. Sections of the person-centred community with strong anti-psychiatry or anti-medical model views may stifle such debate. What may limit such stifling though, is person-centred practitioners' understanding that much of mental health practice is influenced by overwhelming and unreasonable pressures and demands placed on mental health professionals, in response to government policy and rising public expectations. This book tries to give a flavour of some of these pressures. By exploring the person-centred approach in the context of psychiatry, I hope to provide a more effective bridge between two very different worlds that have often eyed each other with mutual suspicion and cynicism.

Third, within the person-centred community, certainly in the UK, there have been moves to explore wider applications of the person-centred approach, i.e. its application beyond therapy. This book is not specifically about therapy (often known as client-centred therapy), but about an approach that can be applied within health care contexts outside therapy relationships. In writing this book I join with Joseph and Worsley who state that 'there are social, political and financial forces operating against the expansion of the Person-Centred Approach, and that the person-centred movement must make its voice heard if it is to continue to make inroads into new territories' (2005, p. 7). I want, therefore, to explore something of what may be involved in practising the person-centred approach within mental health services whilst not practising as a therapist. How, for example, is it possible to practise the person-centred approach when confronted by the overwhelming number, and particular nature, of tasks, goals, responsibilities and relationships mental health professionals are engaged in? This is just one of the many barriers that make my final, and overall, aim of this book perhaps the most ambitious.

Simply, I believe that the dehumanising effects of the NHS mental health system need to be highlighted and addressed. Psychiatry and mental health services need to reappraise their values and philosophy of human beings, mental distress, relationship and helping because, in my opinion, they are failing to provide a sufficiently caring and adequate response to those in need who come into contact with the services. I believe the person-centred approach could contribute powerfully to such a reappraisal and I hope its values can begin to infiltrate a culture that is, in my opinion, in desperate need of them. The ultimate aim of this book is to contribute to a humanising process, even though such an ambition may seem naïve and hopelessly idealistic. I believe that holding on to ideals is important, whilst acknowledging that this may often lead to disappointment and frustration. I realise I am idealistic concerning the kind of health culture and working environment I would like to work in and see available for patients, but I don't think I am blind to constraining factors such as the political and economic realities in the UK.

The author

I believe I am well placed to write a book such as this being, unusually, both a psychiatrist and a person-centred counsellor. For the past eight or so years, from the time I left the NHS for a year to undertake a full-time diploma in counselling in the person-centred approach, I have inhabited the worlds of psychiatry, counselling and the person-centred approach. Although for the past four years I have practised solely as a psychiatrist and not as a counsellor, I did at one time attempt to integrate counselling practice within my psychiatric post. This eventually proved too difficult and was fraught with role conflicts, particularly when my counselling values clashed with the expectations on me as a doctor carrying certain medical responsibilities.

My training in person-centred counselling, rather than other approaches to counselling or psychotherapy, was a highly conscious decision. Whilst I had long held an interest in psychotherapy, I did not wish to train as a therapist within the NHS and not as a specialty within psychiatry, not least because training in the person-centred approach is not on offer within the NHS. I knew it was this approach that most interested me and that fitted most closely to my personal philosophy and values about human beings and helping relationships. I also wanted to distance myself from the NHS culture and from the medical profession, feeling disillusioned, angry and burnt out early on in my psychiatric training. I also realised I did not want to be a 'career psychiatrist', by which I mean I did not want to pursue training to be a consultant, and all that would entail.

I don't remember when I first came across Carl Rogers, but I do remember thinking about some of his ideas whilst I was at medical school and before I knew

I wanted to specialise in psychiatry. It was not only his emphasis on experiencing and communicating certain attitudes towards people that drew me (attitudes which I was in desperate need of receiving myself), but also his ideas about the nature of human beings, personality and mental distress, as well as what human beings need in order to grow and heal. All this contrasted sharply with what I was learning at medical school with its focus on disease processes and the training of doctors to regard patients with detached objectivity. Simply, Rogers and the person-centred approach represented for me a light of hope, as it has done ever since, in a health care culture that is often characterised by so-called 'professional distance', judgemental attitudes, competition amongst professionals and a language of diagnosis and treatment rather than relationships and healing. However, I think it was also what the person-centred approach has to say about the issues of power and expertise that most drew me, being someone who had become aware of and sensitive to power dynamics, particularly in helping contexts. I can see how feelings of powerlessness during my upbringing and from many experiences continuing into my adulthood have contributed to this sensitivity. What has led to my interest in counselling and psychotherapy is also fairly easy to trace and this is where this autobiographical sketch starts to feel somewhat riskier.

My interest in the healing relationship quite simply evolved from my own need for and experience of it. Throughout much of my time at medical school I was depressed, often profoundly. Completing my degree seems rather a miracle and was in part due to taking time out from my course on a couple of occasions (which meant it was seven years before I finally left Southampton University Medical School), and the unfailing generosity of a couple of friends in lending me their lecture notes and generally keeping me in touch with things on the numerous occasions when I couldn't face turning up to lectures and seminars. They were for me harrowing years, characterised by feelings of immense loneliness, desperation and regular questioning of my desire to train as a doctor. I came to detest the competitive culture amongst my fellow students and the preoccupation with power, status and hierarchy for which the medical profession is often noted. However, there was more to it than simply a reaction to an environment and culture in which I didn't feel comfortable. If my self-esteem and inner security were decidedly fragile, the seeds of this were sown during my upbringing. That my parents did their best to provide a loving home for my brother and me, given their circumstances, I have no doubt. Yet, by the time I entered adulthood I was experiencing deep feelings of worthlessness and a painful longing to be understood and feel accepted. It has taken many years of therapy and other supportive relationships and friendships to achieve a good measure of repair. Needless to say, it was experiencing therapists who were genuine and who had a capacity to experience and communicate deep empathy and unconditional acceptance towards me that 'brought me in from the cold' and taught me about the qualities of healing relationships. The transforming power of such relationships cannot be overestimated, in my opinion. Incidentally, I do not believe that such qualities are found only in person-centred or other therapists. I also want to add that for me it was important to choose carefully which therapist I wanted to see and I was prepared to keep myself in financial debt to pay for a form of help there was little chance of receiving on the NHS, unless I was extraordinarily lucky.

Like many helpers then, my motivation for what I do is in large part drawn from my own experiences of being helped. It is not uncommon for people to look for meaning in light of the difficulties and sufferings they experience. For me, meaning is not something to be discovered but something to be given. In other words, doing what I am now doing, including writing this book, is a way of giving meaning to my years of depression and painful questioning (a vulnerability to which I remain predisposed, although less so now). What I have needed to develop over recent years, though, is a sense that my job (or vocation, to use a rather unfashionable concept) and writing are not the only things which give meaning to my life and from which I derive a sense of purpose.

This book is also the fruit of a good deal of questioning and a growing interest in philosophy and ethics, particularly related to psychiatry. For me the person-centred approach, and Carl Rogers especially, enables me to think about the relationship between science and the more personal and subjective aspects of existence. Within the person-centred approach I also find a home for some of my spiritual questioning and journeying, although this is not described in this book. Most of all, I find the person-centred approach provides a reassuring counterblast to a culture that is increasingly alienating and rejecting of individuals as unique persons, and in which one has to compete hard in order to survive.

Structure and style

I want to add here a few notes on how I have structured this book and to say something of its content and style, including various terms I have used.

The final structure has evolved during the two-and-a-half years that I have been writing this book and it has fallen naturally into two main parts. The first part focuses more heavily on theory and philosophy, whilst the second considers the practice of the person-centred approach in the context of mental health settings. There is some overlap of themes and ideas but I have endeavoured to keep this to a minimum and to keep the structure as tight as possible.

In presenting the person-centred approach I have tried to keep in mind both those who have no prior knowledge and understanding of the approach, and also those who have a good knowledge but who might, perhaps, appreciate seeing the theory in a different way. Certainly, thinking about the theory and philosophy of the person-centred approach in the context of psychiatry has deepened my own understanding and has forced me to focus on dimensions I had previously glossed over because I had assumed, wrongly, that I had already grasped them.

I have tried to present ideas and concepts in as simple and accessible a way as possible without being simplistic. In other words, I hope to appeal to both the casual reader, as well as those with more scholarly leanings. I have researched and read widely and this is, I think, reflected in the text and references. Nevertheless, there will inevitably be topics and areas that could have benefited from a more comprehensive coverage or explanation, or perhaps a more solid integration of thoughts and ideas. I consider much of this book to be work in progress.

It is important to point out that the person-centred approach is itself a developing one. I have generally focused on the philosophy and theory as originally described by Rogers and, as such, this book is a presentation of what has been termed the 'classical' (the original) person-centred approach. I also want to say that this book is not an attempt to create a kind of 'meta-theory' in which the theory and philosophy of Rogers become integrated into other theories and practice. Psychiatry is already an eclectic mixture of various schools of thought and practice, although how mental health services and professionals function is largely dictated by political and economic considerations.

As for the political scene, I have tried to integrate an awareness and basic understanding of the UK's political and economic realities throughout various chapters. These aspects of the text will clearly be more relevant to readers in the UK familiar with the NHS and the current Labour government. Nevertheless, I hope my references to UK mental health policy will not be off-putting to readers in other countries and systems of health care, particularly those experiencing similar issues and concerns.

Now follows a little explanation of some of the terms I frequently use. Despite the person-centred approach as applied to counselling and psychotherapy sometimes being known as 'client-centred therapy', my own preference is to use the term 'person-centred therapy'. This is because for me the word 'person' is more meaningful than the term 'client'. Also, it enables a greater acknowledgement of the person of the helper and the fact that there are at least two persons in any encounter. The person-centred approach is also the term Rogers uses to describe the application of the approach outside the therapy relationship and this book is not specifically about counselling or psychotherapy. As for these forms of help, the person-centred approach generally regards counselling and psychotherapy as describing the same activity and therefore tends to use these terms interchangeably. I share this view and I often refer to this form of help simply as 'therapy' and practitioners as 'therapists'. Some discussion on this issue can be found in Chapter 6. I sometimes use the term 'person-centred practitioner' to refer to counsellors, psychotherapists, psychologists or other helpers whose work is orientated towards therapy and whose philosophy and core values are person-centred.

I have often tended to use the term 'psychiatry' rather loosely to refer to mental health settings or the mental health system, even though psychiatry also applies to a branch of Medicine. When I refer to it specifically as a medical specialty I hope I have made this clear. 'Mental health settings' generally refers to specialist 'secondary care', which includes inpatient, outpatient and day patient units, although I recognise that much mental health care occurs within 'primary care' (general practice) settings. Much of this book is therefore relevant to the practice of mental health care whatever the actual location and whichever professional is involved. In keeping with this I use the term 'mental health professional' as a generic term to include psychiatrists, mental health social workers, nurses, psychologists, psychotherapists, occupational therapists, support workers and any helper allied to the mental health professions. When I refer to a particular professional group I have made this clear.

Finally, I want to say something about my tendency to use the term 'patient', even though people coming into contact with mental health services are also variously called 'clients', 'service-users' or, occasionally, 'consumers' or 'survivors'. I am aware how much language matters and how important the issue of naming is in psychiatry. It may be that some person-centred practitioners will feel uncomfortable with my regular use of the term patient. In part, my use of this label is due to habit. In general, doctors tend to use the term patient. People being cared for in hospital also tend to be referred to as patients, whereas in the community the preferred term is often client. These days, the politically correct term is service-user. I must admit that I dislike the term service-user, agreeing with Coulter (2002) that it is a clumsy term, has connotations of drug misuse and does not convey a sense of active partnership. I appreciate that for some, the label patient, particularly within psychiatry, is an emotionally loaded one, with associations of passivity on the part of patients and control and authority on the part of the doctor or other professional. I use the term patient simply to refer to a person receiving medical or other types of care and help. Power imbalances and passivity exist regardless of the terms used, as does stigma. There is also little evidence that the majority of people object to the term patient, at least when used by doctors (Ritchie, Hayes and Ames, 2000; McGuire-Snieckus, McCabe and Priebe, 2003). In contrast, the convention in therapy situations is to use the term client, with which I am comfortable, although I do not use this term often in this book because therapy is not its main focus. My real preference is to use the term 'person'.

The audience

Given my ambitions for this book, as stated earlier, I hope to appeal to as broad a readership as possible. Whilst writing I have often had mental health professionals in mind, including those in training, with no bias towards any particular profession, even though I do draw a lot from my own experience as a psychiatrist. I also hope to appeal to members of the person-centred community, including therapists, supervisors and trainers. Naturally I hope this book is of particular interest to person-centred practitioners with an interest in and experience of working in NHS mental health settings or other health care settings. I hope though, that anyone interested in the values and philosophy of the person-centred approach will find much of interest, as well as people who are concerned, like me, that there is increasing neglect of the importance of relationship and certain listening attitudes in mental health practice. I hope that anyone who shares with me feelings of dismay at the dismissal of values that honour the uniqueness and relational needs of human beings, as well as the quest for a sense of meaning, particularly when in mental distress, will find much of value in this book.

A final introductory note ...

One of the things I experience being both a psychiatrist and person-centred counsellor, i.e. belonging to two camps often in direct opposition, is being caught in the crossfire. I am aware of potential criticisms from within both psychiatry and the person-centred community. From psychiatry I hear the hostile voices of those wedded to the medical model and to reductionist approaches to care. Writing such a book risks professional isolation. From the person-centred community I imagine criticism or suspicion from some quarters that through practising as a psychiatrist I am compromising some of the core values of the person-centred approach. Indeed I am compromising certain principles and values and it feels extremely uncomfortable. However, if this book does manage to stimulate critical thinking, debate and some reappraisal of the values and philosophy from which we work, then my satisfaction will vastly outweigh my discomfort and the personal cost of undertaking this project. Of course, I have in any case hugely gained from the process of writing and integrating much of my thinking and experience as a developing person and professional.

References

Coulter A (2002) *The Autonomous Patient. Ending paternalism in medical care.* The Nuffield Trust, London.

Joseph S and Worsley R (2005) Psychopathology and the Person-Centred Approach: Building Bridges between disciplines. In S Joseph and R Worsley (eds) *Person-Centred Psychopathology. A Positive Psychology of Mental Health.* PCCS Books, Ross-on-Wye, pp. 1–8.

McGuire-Snieckus R, McCabe R and Priebe S (2003) Patient, client or service user? A survey of patient preferences of dress and address of six mental health professions. *Psychiatric Bulletin,* **27**: 305–308.

Ritchie C, Hayes D and Ames D (2000) Patient or client? The opinions of people attending a psychiatric clinic. *Psychiatric Bulletin,* **24**: 447–450.

Section One:

Theoretical and philosophical challenges of the person-centred approach

Chapter 1

What is the person-centred approach?

'The central hypothesis of this approach can be briefly stated. It is that the individual has within himself or herself vast resources for self-understanding, for altering his or her self-concept, attitudes, and self-directed behaviour – and that these resources can be tapped if only a definable climate of facilitative psychological attitudes can be provided.'

(Rogers, 1990/1986, p. 135)

Introduction

Not long ago I saw a job advertisement on an NHS Trust website for a project manager, aiming to attract someone who was 'passionate about ensuring a "person centred" approach to working practice'. I was immediately curious. Was the NHS really looking for someone who, like me, was an advocate of the person-centred approach as formulated by Carl Rogers? Responding to my curiosity, and willing to challenge my scepticism, I replied to the advertisement asking what was meant by the term 'person centred'. My scepticism was confirmed. It was simply a direct reference to Standard Two of the 'National Service Framework for Older People' (DH, 2001). This states that 'older people and their carers should receive person-centred care and services which respect them as individuals and which are arranged around their needs' (p. 23).

The National Service Framework (NSF) for Older People is not the only Department of Health (DH) document that uses the term 'person centred'. More recently, guidance on developing a psychiatric workforce, whose contributors include the Royal College of Psychiatrists and the National Institute for Mental Health in England (NIMHE), refers to providing 'developmentally orientated, person-centred, socially inclusive and recovery-orientated services' (DH, 2004a, p. 6). There has been a veritable proliferation of person-centred terminology within health care settings, but it is rarely used with reference to the person-centred approach as outlined by Carl Rogers, his co-workers and person-centred practitioners today.

This is a significant barrier to promoting an accurate understanding of the person-centred approach in mental health and other NHS settings, making it difficult for person-centred counsellors and psychotherapists to establish themselves and their approach. In this chapter I shall review in more detail some of the ways in which the terms 'person-centred' and the similar sounding terms 'patient-centred' and 'patient-centred care' are used within the NHS and other health care organisations.

However, other major challenges for the person-centred approach are that it runs counter to the prevailing culture within health care organisations, as this book will regularly demonstrate. I also believe that an accurate understanding of the approach rests on an appreciation of its underlying philosophy and values. Put another way, a great deal of misunderstanding and superficial treatment of the approach results from the absence of a basic grasp of its fundamental philosophical principles. It is unfortunate that even graduates of some counselling training courses claiming to have as their core theoretical model the person-centred approach, lack an appreciation of basic philosophical principles. Many mental health professionals are offered even less opportunity to explore the foundation of person-centred theory and practice, receiving only a cursory introduction to the ideas of Carl Rogers and the person-centred approach. Psychiatrists, according to Gask (2004), are not routinely educated in cultural and philosophical concepts at all, let alone the philosophy of the person-centred approach and other humanistic approaches.

In this chapter then, I shall also present the key philosophical principles and values of the person-centred approach. The final section will introduce the major contribution of Carl Rogers and provide an overview of person-centred theory and practice that will be explored in more depth in subsequent chapters.

Patient-centred, person-centred care and the person-centred approach: are you confused?

Uses of the term 'patient-centred'

The terms 'patient centred' and 'patient centred care' are now used frequently in policy documents and guidelines. For example, The NHS Plan states that 'the NHS must be redesigned to be patient centred' (DH, 2000, p. 17). Indeed, developing patient-centred services is a major theme of the current Labour government's health policy. So when health care professionals use the term 'person-centred' do they mean 'patient-centred'?

The situation is confusing. It is often by no means clear what health care professionals and the government mean when they use the term 'patient centred' (with or without a hyphen). In my reading of the health care literature, I have noticed two main ways in which the term is used. First, it is used to describe a value or philosophy of health care (a guiding principle) that informs policy development. The Committee on Quality of Health Care in America (2001) provides an example of this when it gives 'patient centred' as one of six key characteristics of ideal health care. In their report, 'patient centred' refers to respecting and responding to individuals' preferences, needs and values. There are clear similarities here with The NHS Plan, in which one of the core principles of the NHS is described as follows: 'The NHS will shape its services around the needs and preferences of individual patients, their families and their carers' (DH, 2000, p. 3).

The second way in which the term 'patient centred' is used is as a description of the nature of the relationship between a doctor (or other helping professional) and their patient, and of what the doctor–patient consultation should achieve (Schofield, 2000). This is sometimes referred to as 'patient centred medicine'. As a clinical method, this has become an academic subject and also a focus of research. Various forms have been developed in recent years, initially as a reaction to the paternalistic consultation style. Essentially 'patient centred care' represents a change in the mindset of the doctor from the traditional authoritarian and controlling stance, towards one of shared decision-making and patient empowerment (Stewart, Brown, Weston *et al*, 2003). The striving towards partnership between patients and professionals lies at the heart of such care. Built into a 'patient centred consultation' is an attempt on the part of the professional to understand the whole person. 'Patient centred' denotes a focus on the patient rather than the problem or disease. By listening to the patient's perspective, the helper will also develop an understanding of the patient's subjective experience of illness. The conversation will not, in other words, be dominated by the language and process of making a diagnosis. Patient-centred communication skills include active listening and providing empathy and support.

Whilst it is clear what is meant by 'patient-centred' as a clinical method and type of relationship, it is less clear what 'patient-centred' and 'person-centred' mean when describing a value or philosophy of health care. What attitudes and values are actually being referred to? Or are these just convenient, 'feel good' terms that have now become highly favoured by politicians, managers, and those charged with making policy and writing guidelines and mission statements?

The meaning of 'person-centred' within health care settings

The term 'person centred' in UK health policy seems to have undergone changes in its meaning. It now has as its main focus not only the concept of partnership, but also that of patient choice. Furthermore, when referred to by politicians, choice is often wrapped up in the language of consumerism. For example, Prime Minister Blair in 'The NHS Improvement Plan' refers to the public as expecting 'high-quality products, better services, choice and convenience' (DH, 2004b, p. 3), and asserts that the NHS must be modernised accordingly. In The NHS Improvement Plan, patient choice has become linked to providing 'personalised care' when it refers to 'giving people greater personal choice and empowering them to personalise their care to ensure the quality and convenience that they want' (p. 9). In the Executive Summary of The NHS Improvement Plan the words 'personal' or 'personalised' are mentioned no less than 22 times. Thus, 'person centred' comes to be equated with notions of personal and personalised care, and seems to represent an ideology in which consumerism, choice, 'plurality of provision' of services, and market forces are viewed as the drivers of health care delivery in the public as well as private sector. In addition to being linked to choice, 'person centred' and 'patient-centred' services describe services that are interested in giving patients more say through patient surveys and the development of strategies for patient and public involvement in service planning.

In the academic literature of the helping professions, the term 'person-centred' is often used to convey humanistic ideas in general. For Barker (2003) 'person-centred care' means focusing on the person – the human being – rather than the pathology. It conveys attitudes of respect for the individual with his or her unique experience and needs. For Watkins (2001), 'person-centred' conveys a holistic approach, particularly with reference to the assessment of mental health problems. Watkins also uses the term 'person-centred' with reference to Carl Rogers, but like many other authors, misses the full distinctiveness and radical nature of the person-centred approach. For example, the non-directive nature of the person-centred approach is not emphasised. Watkins and Barker provide good examples in mental health literature of authors who refer to the person-centred approach when in fact they are describing the broad sweep of humanistic ideas and philosophy, or simply notions of holistic care. A gross example of the misleading use of the term 'person-centred approach' can be found in the title of a book that has nothing to do with the person-centred approach of Carl Rogers. 'Psychotherapy with Suicidal People: A Person Centred Approach' (Leenaars, 2004) is simply concerned with developing a holistic approach to suicidal ideation.

It should now be clear why it is impossible to formulate a definition of 'person-centred' as applied in health care settings. The best one can do is to generate a list of possible meanings or concepts with which it is associated.

The person-centred approach in health care settings

Despite the wide use of the term 'person centred', both in mental health and other health care settings, it is rare, in my experience, for it to be used with direct reference to the person-centred approach as a major theoretical system, philosophy and practice developed by Carl Rogers, his co-workers and practitioners of person-centred counselling and psychotherapy today. Perhaps this is unsurprising given the fact that it is mainly counsellors and psychotherapists who are likely to study this approach in depth. Training courses for many mental health professionals will usually include on their curriculum something about Carl Rogers and the person-centred approach, but in recent years 'skills-based' approaches such as that of Gerard Egan (1994), cognitive-behavioural approaches, and approaches that lend themselves more easily to measurement, structured working and evidence-based practice, feature more heavily.

There are many aspects of the kinds of person-centred and patient-centred care just described that person-centred counsellors and psychotherapists will recognise. Carl Rogers and the development of person-centred therapy from the middle of the last century have undoubtedly been massively influential in the helping professions. Sometimes the influence of Rogers is acknowledged, for example in the development of the patient-centred clinical method by Stewart, Brown, Weston et al (2003). More often than not though, the term 'person centred' is used loosely and without an understanding of where its ideas and philosophy have originated. Worse is when the term is used simply as a catchphrase with no particular meaning. Sometimes it simply seems to be a term of political correctness.

Advocates of the person-centred approach often struggle to explain their way of working and make a claim for its distinctive and radical nature. The widespread and varying use of person-centred terms is a significant impediment that makes it even more essential for person-centred practitioners to be rigorous in checking their own use of language and terminology, and to be clear about what they mean and what they want to convey. It also doesn't help that some therapists describe themselves as person-centred when their actual practice reveals that they have departed from the fundamental values of the person-centred approach and consists of an eclectic mixture of techniques, thus misrepresenting the person-centred approach. It is also necessary for the person-centred practitioner, in attempting to explain their way of working, to check what the listener has understood, since adherents of the medical model may find it difficult to comprehend an approach that adopts an altogether different paradigm.

More than a type of therapy

The person-centred approach is most often associated with a type of counselling or psychotherapy. This is understandable since Rogers and his colleagues spent much of their working lives as therapists, and much of what Rogers writes is in the context of therapy. Furthermore, most texts with 'person-centred' in the title, academic or otherwise, are concerned with the approach as it relates specifically to counselling and psychotherapy.

It is, however, becoming increasingly recognised that, whilst the person-centred approach may have originated as a very distinctive type of therapy, revolutionary even, it is also an 'approach to life both in and beyond therapy', as described by Embleton-Tudor *et al* (2004, p. 3) in their recent book 'The Person-Centred Approach. A Contemporary Introduction'. In this book the person-centred approach is further described as 'a comprehensive, coherent and holistic approach to human life and concerns' (p. 3). In other words, it can be applied to all aspects of life and living, and this book is one of the first post-Rogers to examine the person-centred approach to aspects of life and living outside therapy.

Rogers himself recognises that the person-centred approach can be embraced outside the therapy room when he writes '... I am no longer talking simply about psychotherapy, but about a point of view, a philosophy, an approach to life, a way of being ...' (1980, p. xvii). It is recognition of this that leads him to use the term 'person-centred approach' where previously he and his colleagues would always have referred to 'client-centred therapy'.

What Rogers formulates is a philosophy of human beings and relationships 'which fits any situation in which *growth* – of a person, a group, or a community – is part of the goal' (Rogers, 1980, p. xvii). This means that the person-centred approach can be taken into any situation involving human beings. It can therefore be viewed, in Rogers' words, as a '*philosophy* of living and relationships' (1980, pp. 37–38, original italics), or as 'a practical philosophy of living' (Van Kalmthout, 2004, p. 197). Van Kalmthout is keen to highlight the approach as a philosophy to be *lived* rather than one just to intellectualise. Specific fields outside therapy to which Rogers devoted his energies, particularly in his later years, include group work, leadership, international peace work (realising his ideas had powerful political implications), and the fields of education and learning. In addition, many have testified to how Rogers embodied the person-centred approach in the way he lived his life and related to others, in both his personal and professional life.

For me, the person-centred approach also involves entering the challenging terrain of ethics and values. Ethics is essentially concerned with morals and values. A summary definition of values is that they are 'conceptions of the morally desirable' (New, 2002, p. 20). Living the person-centred approach certainly involves embracing a set of values. The approach can therefore be described as an ethical engagement with life, living and relationships. I also regard this as much more than working from a professional, ethical code of practice to which most health professionals are required to subscribe, since clearly I am again referring to the approach as one that can be lived outside the workplace. Put another way, the values with which I live my life are also those I bring to my work.

As a psychiatrist I am conscious daily of the ethical issues that confront me. As someone who also tries to embrace the person-centred approach, I experience these ethical issues as another layer of complexity. The values to which I aspire often seem to be in direct conflict with those of mainstream psychiatry and the organisation within which I work. Attitudes towards 'risk management' and beliefs about the right for self-determination are just two examples, as is the value the person-centred approach places on the quality of relating and attitudes towards human beings. However, outside my job I am conscious also of how much the philosophy and values of the person-centred approach come into conflict with those of modern western society. The person-centred approach does not sit comfortably within our culture, dominated as it is by materialist values, the quest for efficiency, cost-effectiveness and hitting targets. Quality, authenticity and intimacy of relating and relationship, for which so many people deeply yearn, are jeopardised by the values of modern western culture. This results in increasing levels of desperation and loneliness within our homes and communities. Living the person-centred approach and embracing it as a 'way of being' – a phrase Rogers makes famous both in and outside the therapy context and work place – pose an immense challenge for the person who takes seriously his or her beliefs and values concerning who we are as human beings and how we relate to one another.

The philosophical values of the person-centred approach

'The person-centred approach, then, is primarily a way of being that finds its expression in attitudes and behaviours that create a growth-promoting climate. It is a basic philosophy rather than simply a technique or method. When this philosophy is lived, it helps the person expand the development of his or her own capacities. When it is lived, it also stimulates constructive change in others.'

(Rogers, 1990/1986, p. 138)

When Rogers developed his understanding of persons and a theory of therapy, he challenged with radical ideas the professional circles of his day. Behavioural and psychoanalytical psychologies were the two dominant schools of thought within the academic and clinical worlds of psychology and psychiatry. Psychoanalysis, although a 'broad church', often emphasises pathology, whilst behaviourism is concerned with behaviours that can be viewed mechanistically and objectively.

The person-centred approach is commonly associated with humanistic psychology. Humanistic psychology is described by Abraham Maslow (1908–1970), one of the most prominent humanistic thinkers, as 'third force psychology', providing an alternative to the first two psychological approaches of psychoanalysis and behaviourism. The view that a human being 'is positive in nature – is basically socialised, forward-moving, rational and realistic' (Rogers, 1967, p. 91) stands in stark contrast to the 'bad animal' view of human nature often postulated by psychoanalysis, particularly Freudian schools. Humanistic psychology though, rather than being a single, organised, theoretical system, is a school of many ideas from a great variety of thinkers, both when it was developing as a new movement in the 1960s, and currently.

Humanistic psychology should not be confused with secular humanism, although it often is. An academic paper in a journal on nurse education by Purdy (1997) provides just one example, confusing the terms in its very title – 'Humanist ideology and nurse education'. Likewise, Pilgrim in 'Key Concepts in Mental Health' refers to 'Humanism' as a type of psychological approach (2005, p. 97). Humanism and humanistic psychology couldn't be more different. Whilst humanistic psychology is often open to exploration of the spiritual and trans-personal realms and very open to the world of emotions, central to humanism is a rejection of religious belief, spiritual and supernatural ideas. Humanism promotes human reason and rationality.

Some key ideas and values within humanistic psychology are included in the following descriptions:

- it 'emphasises especially the creative, constructive, aesthetic and aspirational qualities of human nature and human beings' (Embleton-Tudor *et al*, 2004, p. 22);
- it is concerned with the 'uniqueness of the individual, the quest for values and meaning, and the freedom inherent in self-direction and self-fulfilment' (Hjelle and Ziegler, 1992, p. 485);
- it recognises that in all life forms there is 'a tendency towards more complex organisation' and in humans 'the fulfilment of potential and the actualisation of the "self", the process of becoming all of which we are capable' (Tudor and Merry, 2002, p. 68).

Key tenets of humanistic psychology include its more positive and optimistic view of human nature, what motivates us and what we may become, i.e. it focuses on potentials. Each individual's subjective experience is considered unique. Human beings are regarded as intrinsically good with the capacity for love and compassion, although their capacity for behaving antisocially and committing evil acts is not denied either. Concepts of love, creativity, growth and spirituality are topics of particular interest in humanistic psychology. Further-more, in contrast to traditional scientific viewpoints, humanistic psychology forms an integrated view of human beings rather than selecting parts to look at that 'reduce' the person. In other words, it is holistic rather than reductionistic.

Humanistic psychology and the person-centred approach also draw on two other philosophical approaches, which I shall briefly describe. These are exist-entialism and phenomenology, the latter being a development of existentialism.

Existentialism largely grew out of the thinking of Søren Kierkegaard (1813–1855). The other existentialist philosopher whose thinking appealed to Rogers is Martin Buber (1878–1965), who was also a theologian. Rogers quotes both Kierkegaard and Buber in his writings. As with humanistic psychology, an overarching definition of existentialism is difficult to formulate, but the main concepts that influence Rogers and which inform the person-centred approach are:

- having freedom and choice to decide who we are, how we behave and the right to self-determination;

- having the ability to take personal responsibility for decision making and for our actions;
- its emphasis on subjective reality and regarding human behaviour as the result of our perception of ourselves and our surroundings;
- its interest in how individuals construe meaning from experience;
- how it relates to the idea that 'knowledge' depends on the approach and nature of the 'knower'.

However, whilst Rogers readily embraces the more positive aspects of existentialism such as freedom and individuality, possibly reflecting the American pioneering spirit and his own cultural background, he does not readily embrace the limitations and the 'tragic dimensions of existence' (Yalom, 1980, p. 19), which other existentialist thinkers focused upon, especially European existentialists such as Jean-Paul Sartre (1905–1980). The Europeans' preoccupation with human anguish, despair, and the limitations imposed by death and isolation, do not sit comfortably with Rogers (Tudor and Worrall, 2006) and do not easily align themselves with mainstream person-centred philosophy today.

Phenomenology is a term that will perhaps be more familiar to mental health professionals than existentialism. However, the phenomenological influences on the person-centred approach should not be confused with the usual meaning of the term in psychiatric settings, although even within psychiatry the term can be used in different ways. The laziest use of the term in psychiatry is simply as a synonym for symptoms and signs, i.e. mental phenomena. More precisely, it is viewed as a method deployed by psychiatrists and other mental health professionals involving, according to Sims (2003) 'the observation and categorisation of abnormal psychological events, the internal experiences of the patient and his consequent behaviour' (p. 3). The method is one of using empathy to explore the patient's subjective world. In psychiatric settings though, empathy is often very simplistically understood (the person-centred understanding of empathy is presented in Chapter 8). Within psychiatry, Karl Jaspers (1883–1969), a psychiatrist, is the person most commonly associated with the development of phenomenology.

The philosophical system of phenomenology that influences Rogers is based on the thinking of Edmund Husserl (1859–1938), Martin Heidegger (1889–1976) and Maurice Merleau-Ponty (1907–1961). Whilst this system is concerned with the patient's subjective experience, the similarity with Jaspers and the psychiatric use of the term seems to end here. It is primarily interested in how human beings perceive, experience and give meaning to the world around them. According to Embleton-Tudor *et al* (2004) 'it suggests that "reality" is not fixed, out there and objective, but that it depends to a large extent on our perception of it, which is in turn informed by whatever biases, prejudices and perceptual filters we bring to it' (p. 18).

For Rogers it is the way reality is perceived that matters, and the fact that we behave according to our subjective realities. Thorne (2003) also points out that this phenomenological attitude may be directly linked to a belief in the fundamental worth of human beings, stating that 'such an approach takes as its basic assumption that a person's subjective experience is worthy of the deepest respect even if to others it may appear bizarre or misguided' (p. 24).

In highlighting humanistic psychology and philosophy I want to encourage deeper reflection on those values and ideas which many professionals find superficially attractive, but readily abandon in favour of the more dominant philosophies and ideologies within the mental health culture. It is regrettable that when concepts such as human beings' uniqueness, quest for meaning, self-direction and self-fulfilment do resonate with mental health professionals, they do not translate into clinical practice. Sacrifice of such values is often simply because of the seemingly greater importance and priority attached to risk assessments, prescribing medication, formulating care plans, form filling and generally responding to the demands of the prevailing political and economic agendas.

Patients are likely to receive many confusing and conflicting messages when they come into contact with mental health professionals. UK mental health policy is a rich source of ideological contradiction and conflict. Another source of confusion is the number of different mental health professions working from different theoretical perspectives. In the first instance, simply being aware of the many competing philosophies and values, and the confusion and tensions this creates, would at least be a good basis for entering dialogue and debate with colleagues, managers and politicians. Having some philosophical grounding would facilitate such awareness. How often do we ask ourselves what it is that we really believe in? Further, how important is it to us to stick by our values in our daily practice, or at least to try?

The main features of person-centred theory and practice

In this final section I want to introduce the main features of the person-centred approach. In particular, I want to highlight those aspects of the approach that represent what has come to be known as the 'classical' position, i.e. the original theory as presented by Rogers. What follows is only a brief summary of the main features, since they will be covered in more depth in subsequent chapters. It also needs to be stated that the theory and ideas of Rogers, and other person-centred theorists and prominent practitioners, are more comprehensively covered elsewhere in literature exclusively dedicated to the person-centred approach. The further reading section at the end of this chapter lists some of the major texts, as well as Rogers' most well known writings.

Rogers' main theoretical interests

Rogers is often more known for his ideas on therapy and the formulation of the conditions within therapy that lead to constructive personality change. Yet his theory of therapy relates to a comprehensive and integrated theory of personality and behaviour that not only considers how healthy personalities develop, but also what constitutes and contributes to psychological disturbance. His most comprehensive theory statement is usually considered to be 'A Theory of Therapy, Personality and Interpersonal Relationships as Developed in the Client-Centred Framework' (1959). This not only details his theory of personality, a key concept of which is commonly termed the 'actualising tendency' (or alternatively, the organism's tendency to actualise). This statement represents one of Rogers' major contributions to the world of counselling and psychotherapy. It outlines six conditions (described in Chapter 7) which, if present, will lead to constructive personality change. These conditions, hypothesised by Rogers as both 'necessary and sufficient', include what is commonly known today as the three 'core conditions' of congruence, unconditional positive regard and empathy. Rogers also postulates what he terms the 'fully functioning person' (described more fully in Chapter 2). Simply, the fully functioning person is a 'person-in-process' rather than one who has arrived, and which he describes as 'synonymous with optimal psychological adjustment, optimal psychological maturity, complete congruence, complete openness to experience . . .' (1959, p. 235).

Thus, Rogers is both a personality theorist and a theorist concerning the process of therapy. Furthermore, his ideas are not developed in the abstract. He develops his theory of personality and behaviour through clinical practice and experience as a therapist.

Core principles

In light of developments in theory and in practice in recent years, and the existence of different schools of thought within the person-centred approach, attempts have been made to identify the core principles of the approach and to agree on which aspects deserve the most emphasis. Sanders proposes what he terms 'primary principles' (2004, p. 155). These are:

- the primacy of the actualising tendency which, according to Rogers, is 'the inherent tendency of the organism to develop all its capacities in ways which serve to maintain or enhance the organism' (1959, p. 196), and which is described by Tudor and Merry as 'the sole motivation for human development and behaviour' (2002, p. 3).
- that the six therapeutic conditions are necessary and sufficient (described in Chapter 7). In other words, no other conditions are necessary for constructive personality change. This clearly makes the *relationship* the agent for change.
- the primacy of the non-directive attitude. This attitude (described further in Chapter 5) relates to placing trust in the capacity and tendency of individuals to actualise, given the optimal environment. It is also associated with the person-centred stance on issues of power and expertise.

The attitude towards power has led to the person-centred approach being regarded as radically different from other types of therapy, including therapies within the humanistic tradition. Wilkins is 'doubtful that the principle characteristic of person-centred therapy is its "humanistic" nature', seeing 'its key characteristic as the eschewing of power and expertise' (2003, p. 26). Bozarth (1998) refers to the person-centred approach as a 'revolutionary paradigm'. For him the actualising tendency is the 'foundation block' of therapy, which means that the power rests in the client and the therapist avoids all control over the client and their process. This clearly involves an extraordinary trust in the client and in the potential of human beings to grow, heal and find their own path towards psychological health, given the right conditions.

Given the developments of the approach and the existence of different forms of person-centred therapy such as the 'experiential', 'existential' and 'focusing-orientated' therapies (which has led Margaret Warner (2000) to refer to the many 'tribes' within the 'nation' of the person-centred approach), is it possible to speak of *the* person-centred approach? Like many approaches it is what people claim it to be for themselves. Yet whilst debate is healthy and Rogers himself wanted the approach to develop, in other respects such disagreements about the core features of the approach are unfortunate. They can make it hard for person-centred practitioners to feel secure in their identity when it is already a challenge to make themselves understood within the current health care culture. And 'in the current political and social situation, it is very important that we know exactly what constitutes the true nature of our approach, what we are and what we are not' (Van Kalmthout, 2004, p. 195). I agree.

Research

The two areas of Rogers' work that this book focuses on are his theory of personality and his theory of therapy and helping relationships. What I shall not be covering is one of his other major contributions, that of research. However, it is worth mentioning that as an empirical scientist Rogers is keen always to test his theories and it is hard not to be impressed by his pioneering research efforts. He is one of the first therapists to record therapy sessions, and this well before the digital era, making it an impressive practical achievement. He is keen to evaluate therapist–client interactions in order to understand more fully what is effective about the process of therapy. In addition, he is, as Thorne puts it, 'determined to rescue psychotherapy from those who, for their own reasons, wished to wrap it in mystery and that far from trading on secrecy and mystification it should be revealed in all its observable dimensions' (2003, p. 46).

Conclusion

Whilst debates will continue as to what constitutes the key aspects of the person-centred approach in the field of therapy, wider debates are needed regarding what aspects of the person-centred approach can be developed and applied in other settings, outside the therapy context. There are certainly many challenging questions concerning the person-centred approach within psychiatric settings. For example, what does 'necessary and sufficient' mean regarding the conditions for personality change, in theory and in practice? What are the implications for the non-directive attitude within psychiatric settings? What role does medication have? Where does mental health legislation fit in? How much can I trust in the inherent tendency of a person to actualise when they are acutely and severely mentally disturbed?

Whilst the person-centred approach to therapy, both its theory and practice, is continuing to evolve, likewise the approach outside therapy has much scope for development. This is certainly what Rogers envisages when he writes, 'From its inception, the orientation that has come to be called client-centred psychotherapy has been noted for its growing, changing, developing quality. It has not been a fixed or rigid school of thought' (1990, p. 9).

In terms of encouraging interdisciplinary dialogue, it is probably fair to say that, within psychiatry, the person-centred approach is more likely to appeal to mental health professionals who are more philosophically minded, for whom the quality of relationships with patients has particular emphasis in their work and who value holistic perspectives. Those with a strong ethical base, who are keen to promote the importance of values and values-based practice, are also more likely to join in the debate about what the person-centred approach has to offer and how it can be applied within psychiatric settings.

References

Barker P (2003) Person-centred care: the need for diversity. In Phil Barker (ed) *Psychiatric and Mental Health Nursing. The craft of caring.* Arnold, London, pp. 3–9.

Bozarth J (1998) *Person-Centred Therapy: A Revolutionary Paradigm.* PCCS Books, Ross-on-Wye.

Committee on Quality of Health Care in America (2001) *Crossing the quality chasm: a new health system for the 21st century.* National Academy Press, Washington, DC.

Department of Health (2000) *The NHS Plan. A Plan for Investment. A Plan for Reform.* Department of Health, London.

Department of Health (2001) *National Service Framework for Older People.* Department of Health, London.

Department of Health (National Steering Group) (2004a) *Guidance on New Ways of Working for Psychiatrists in a Multi-disciplinary and Multi-agency Context. Interim Report.* Department of Health, London.

Department of Health (2004b) *The NHS Improvement Plan.* Department of Health, London.

Egan G (1994) *The Skilled Helper. A Problem-Management Approach to Helping.* Brooks/Cole Publishing Company, California.

Embleton-Tudor L, Keemar K, Tudor K *et al* (2004) *The Person-Centred Approach. A Contemporary Introduction.* Palgrave Macmillan, Basingstoke.

Gask L (2004) *A Short Introduction to Psychiatry.* Sage Publications, London.

Hjelle L and Ziegler D (1992) *Personality Theories: Basic Assumptions, Research and Applications.* McGraw-Hill, New York

Leenaars A (2004) *Psychotherapy with Suicidal People: A Person Centred Approach.* Wiley, Chichester.

New B (2002) Thinking about values. In B New and J Neuberger (eds) *Hidden Assets. Values and decision-making in the NHS.* King's Fund, London, pp. 17–30.

Pilgrim D (2005) *Key Concepts in Mental Health.* Sage, London.

Purdy M (1997) Humanist ideology and nurse education. 1. Humanist educational theory. *Nurse Education Today,* **17**: 192–195.

Rogers C (1959) A theory of therapy, personality, and interpersonal relationships, as developed in the client-centred framework. In S Koch (ed) *Psychology: a study of a science. Study 1. Volume 3. Formulations of the person and the social context.* McGraw-Hill, New York, pp. 184–256.

Rogers C (1967) *On Becoming a Person. A therapist's view of psychotherapy.* Constable, London.

Rogers C (1980) *A Way of Being.* Houghton Mifflin, Boston, MA.

Rogers C (1990) A Client-centred/Person-centred Approach to Therapy. In H Kirschenbaum and VL Henderson (eds) *The Carl Rogers Reader.* Constable, London, pp. 135–152. (Original work published 1986)

Rogers C (1990) Client-Centred Therapy. In H Kirschenbaum and VL Henderson (eds) *Carl Rogers: Dialogues.* Constable, London, pp. 9–38.

Sanders P (2004) Mapping person-centred approaches to counselling and psychotherapy. In P Sanders (ed) *The tribes of the person-centred nation.* PCCS Books, Ross-on-Wye, pp. 149–163.

Schofield T (2000) Patient-centred Consultations. *Medicine,* **28(10)**: 22–24.

Sims A (2003) *Symptoms in the Mind. An Introduction to Descriptive Psychopathology.* Saunders, London.

Stewart M, Brown JB, Weston WW *et al* (2003) *Patient-Centred Medicine. Transforming the Clinical Method.* Radcliffe Medical Press, Oxford.

Thorne B (2003) *Carl Rogers.* Sage, London.

Tudor K and Merry T (2002) *Dictionary of Person-Centred Psychology.* Whurr, London.

Tudor K and Worrall M (2006) *Person-Centred Therapy. A Clinical Philosophy.* Routledge, Hove.

Van Kalmthout (2004) Person-Centred Psychotherapy as a Modern System of Meaning. *Person-Centred and Experiential Psychotherapies.* **3**(3): 192–206.

Warner M (2000) Person-centred Psychotherapy: One Nation, Many Tribes. *Person-Centred Journal,* **7**(1): 28–39.

Watkins P (2001) *Mental Health Nursing: the art of compassionate care.* Butterworth Heinemann, Edinburgh.

Wilkins P (2003) *Person-Centred Therapy in Focus.* Sage, London.

Yalom I (1980) *Existential Psychotherapy.* Basic Books, New York.

Further reading

On the Person-Centred Approach, particularly theory and philosophy

- *Dictionary of Person-Centred Psychology* – Tudor and Merry, 2002. Whurr.
- *Invitation to Person-Centred Psychology* – Merry, 1994. Wiley.
- *The Person-Centred Approach. A Contemporary Introduction.* Embleton-Tudor *et al.*, 2004. Palgrave Macmillan.
- *Person-Centred Therapy. A Clinical Philosophy* – Tudor and Worrall, 2006. Routledge.

On Person-Centred Counselling and Psychotherapy

- *Person-Centred Counselling in Action* (2nd edition) – Mearnes and Thorne, 1999. Sage.
- *Learning and Being in Person-Centred Counselling* – Merry, 1999. PCCS.
- *Skills in Person-Centred Counselling and Psychotherapy* – Tolan, 2003. Sage.

On Carl Rogers

- *Carl Rogers* (2e) – Thorne, 2003. Sage.

By Carl Rogers

- *Client-Centred Therapy: Its Current Practice, Implications and Theory.* Rogers, 1951. Constable.
- *On Becoming A Person. A Therapist's View of Psychotherapy.* Rogers, 1967. Constable.
- *The Carl Rogers Reader.* Kirschenbaum and Henderson (eds), 1990. Constable.

Chapter 2

A theory of personality and behaviour

'Of all the problems that have faced human beings since the dawn of recorded history, perhaps the most puzzling has been the riddle of our own nature.'

(Hjelle and Ziegler, 1992, p. 1)

Introduction

In this chapter I present the theory of personality and behaviour as developed by Carl Rogers. In this theory, written in the form of nineteen propositions (1951), Rogers also considers the development of psychological disturbance. In so doing, he presents a model of understanding that challenges the more usual ways of explaining mental distress in psychiatric settings.

One of the core theoretical concepts of Rogers' personality theory is the 'actualising tendency'. His theory also considers the human being as an active, growth-oriented 'organism' (and is therefore sometimes referred to as an 'organismic theory'), although his ideas about and references to the 'self' are also significant. The self is seen as a differentiated part of the whole organism. However, it is worth pointing out that different ways of thinking about some of Rogers' key concepts have emerged over the years. It is also worth noting that Rogers does not define personality as such. Nor for that matter, according to Schmid (1998), does he define the 'person', other than acknowledging the social connotations of the term rather than simply the biological ones of the term organism. Schmid, in the same chapter, has gone on to develop a person-centred understanding of the person. Rogers' theory focuses more on the nature of personality development from our earliest years, and the potential for later change and adaptation. He is more interested in the *process* of development and change.

As a final introductory comment, one of the aspects of Rogers' theory I appreciate is the tentative and non-dogmatic way in which he presents it. He makes clear that his theoretical formulations are hypotheses. I think there is an essential humility and open-mindedness here that many psychologists, psychiatrists, researchers and other mental health professionals could do well to emulate when theorising why such and such person presents with symptom X or problem Y.

The 'organism' and the 'self'

Concepts of the 'self' can be slippery, which is perhaps rather surprising given how many 'self'-related words there are. Indeed, Rogers tells us that at first he considered it a 'vague, ambiguous, scientifically meaningless term' (1959,

p. 200). However, in his work with clients he notices how often they referred to their 'self', or 'me' or 'I', as a significant aspect of their experience as if it were a distinct entity. It is therefore, to him, something that cannot be ignored. As a psychiatrist, I too regularly encounter people wanting and struggling to find ways of expressing their 'self'. I hear questions such as 'who is the real me?' and statements like 'I don't know who I am any more' or 'I just wish I could truly be me'. Talking about the 'self' is often also very painful for many of the people I see, especially when they allude to some 'ideal self' they long to be, or speak of a desperate desire not to be the 'self' they perceive themselves to be.

People also often refer to the self as something static and fixed. However, Wilkins points out that Rogers' conception of the self is as a 'process rather than a fixed entity' (2003, p. 31). This is important because one of the characteristics of the person-centred approach is the emphasis on human beings' capacity to change and develop – of constantly being in a process of 'becoming'. Other terms person-centred practitioners use when referring to the self are 'fluid' and 'dynamic'. This process model of personality development stands in contrast to 'stage theories' such as Sigmund Freud's psychosexual, or Erik Erikson's psychosocial, stages of development. Like other psychologists, such as Freud, Rogers acknowledges the significance of childhood experiences in shaping the personality. Yet for him there is a much greater capacity for personality change later in life than most other personality theorists and many mental health professionals acknowledge. This clearly influences person-centred perspectives on treatment and prognosis.

One misunderstanding that sometimes arises is to regard the person-centred approach as a 'self-psychology'. This is understandable given that notions of the self do feature in Rogers' personality theory. It is certainly true that Rogers regularly refers to the self in his work and writings, but, as I have already noted, he is interested in the human being as a whole organism, which means the whole of our functioning – our biological, cognitive, emotional and behavioural aspects – and the importance of the environment in relation to these. The self, in Rogers' theory, is only that aspect which the organism is conscious of and can reflect upon, i.e. self is akin to self-awareness. Here is another departure from psycho-analytical theory, where notions of the self usually include ideas about the unconscious. What is usually known as self-psychology stems from the work of psychoanalyst Heinz Kohut who sought to revise psychoanalytic theory, placing the concept of self at the centre of his theory, whereas Rogers' theory is more accurately an 'organismic psychology'. Tudor and Worrall (2006) are keen to stress the centrality of the organism, rather than the self, in Rogers' theory, pointing out that this makes it a holistic theory of many parts interacting with each other.

A further difficulty when talking about Rogers' concept of the self is the ease with which many people in western societies associate it with ideas and terms such as 'self-centred', 'selfish' or 'self-worship'. One of the criticisms levelled at the person-centred approach is that it feeds into the 'me culture' and promotes individualism. These days it can be difficult to talk about our 'self' without fear of meeting accusations of being wrapped up in it.

Rogers' personality theory then, hypothesises how human beings develop a concept of self, what constitutes the self, how the personality, through the experiences of the person, becomes disturbed, and finally, the nature of the disturbance. He also hypothesises those characteristics that make up a psychologically healthy person. I shall return to these shortly after attending to one of the key concepts in Rogers' theory of personality – the actualising tendency.

The 'actualising tendency'

I think it is worthy of note that I cannot recall ever once having had a conversation about the actualising tendency with any of my psychiatric colleagues. If I had I am sure I would have remembered it. Yet perhaps it is this tendency that brings many people to seek the help of mental health and other health services; that is the reason why 'time heals'; and is the energy that inspires people to create great works of art, or achieve amazing feats of physical endurance? For Bozarth, the actualising tendency is no less than 'the foundation block of person-centred therapy' (1998, p. 27), and Rogers regards it as 'an underlying basis of the person-centred approach' (1980, p. 119). Here is one of Rogers' descriptions of the actualising tendency:

> '... the inherent tendency of the organism to develop all its capacities in ways which serve to maintain or enhance the organism. It involves not only the tendency to meet what Maslow terms "deficiency needs" for air, food, water, and the like, but also more generalized activities. It involves development toward the differentiation of organs and of functions, expansion in terms of growth, expansion of effectiveness through the use of tools, expansion and enhancement through reproduction. It is development toward autonomy and away from heteronomy, or control by external forces' (1959, p. 196).

Thus, it is in the very nature of the organism (not just the self) to actualise. In addition, Rogers considers this tendency to be the one and only motivator of human development and behaviour concerned with maintaining as well as enhancing the individual. In other words, it encompasses all other drives and motivations – biological, psychological and social – and is a unified and integrated process. He sees an individual drive, such as thirst or hunger, or drive to relate to others, as just one expression of this overarching motivation or tendency that serves to maintain the individual.

Here is another description of the tendency to actualise from Rogers:

> 'I have found that when man is truly free to become what he most deeply is, free to actualize his nature as an organism capable of awareness, then he clearly appears to move toward wholeness and integration' (1990/ 1959, p. 27).

Rogers acknowledges that many psychologists, philosophers and scientists held similar ideas concerning some sort of fundamental, growthful, goal-directed force in nature, even though these ideas are also the fruits of his own observations and clinical practice. He also goes further and describes a 'formative tendency' of the universe, believing that there is a tendency towards increased order and complexity (syntropy as opposed to entropy), and that all things are interconnected.

The actualising tendency is a manifestation of this formative tendency – the part specific to organic life. The tendency towards order and coherence does suggest an intelligent design or purpose, but Rogers does not speculate on the origins of a formative tendency.

Whilst the term 'actualising tendency' is commonly used, Tudor and Worrall point out that this is misleading because it suggests an entity – a 'thing'. They say that it would be more accurate and helpful to say that the organism has a tendency to actualise, or even more accurately, to say that an 'organism *is* a tendency to actualise' (2006, p. 87).

Rogers' hypothesis of the organism's tendency to actualise is a biological one and not a moral one. The tendency is neither good nor bad, it just *is*. Our genetic inheritance is also acknowledged to have an influence. The uniqueness of our genetic code will in fact determine the unique expression of the actualising tendency. In terms of the development of the physical organism in the animal kingdom, the actualising tendency is, for example, responsible for the growth and differentiation of internal organs and their functions. For human beings it is responsible for much more, such as the development of personality, and that which guides and motivates human behaviour. It expresses itself in the social world and its basic direction is towards constructive social behaviour. Thus, the actualising tendency can be said to be a 'pro-social' one. The tendency in humans to actualise, then, encompasses all aspects of our existence and identity – our physical, psychological (emotional and cognitive) and social natures. Many of us would also include the existence in human beings of a spiritual nature to be under the influence of the actualising tendency.

The key question for those in the helping professions is this: given that there is this constructive force – this tendency to actualise – why are we not more perfect physically and mentally? Why do we develop 'unhealthy' patterns of thinking? Why do we behave in destructive ways? Why does there seem to be so much chaos and atrocity in the world, such as the constant threat of global terrorism? Why are there conditions that are described as personality disorder or mental illness? Surely it cannot all be attributed to genetic mishap or brain damage pre- or post-natally? In Rogers' theory this is where the environment needs to be given important consideration. The existence of a tendency to actualise is no guarantor of perfect health because the environment interacts with it for good or ill. In unfavourable, inadequate or destructive conditions, whilst the tendency leads to a striving for the best outcome, a distortion takes place, or as Rogers puts it, the tendency can become 'thwarted or warped' (1980, p. 118). In terms of the human personality, this can result in 'abnormal' or destructive behaviours. However, in keeping with his biological interests and observations of the natural world, Rogers offers a helpful and simple analogy from the plant kingdom that I think is worth quoting. I also find the following passage, in which he is referring to potatoes growing towards a small light source in a dark cellar, inspiring.

'The conditions were unfavorable, but the potatoes would begin to sprout pale white sprouts, so unlike the healthy green shoots they sent up when planted in the soil in the spring. But these sad, spindly sprouts would grow two or three feet in length as they reached toward the distant light of the window. The sprouts were, in their bizarre, futile growth, a sort of desperate expression of the directional tendency I have been describing. They would never become plants, never mature, never fulfill their real potential. But under the most adverse circumstances, they were striving to become. Life would not give up, even if it could not flourish' (1980, p. 118).

The development of personality and the 'self-concept'

In this section I return to the concept of 'self' as hypothesised by Rogers and look at it in more detail, particularly its development. This will include describing the 'self-concept', a term Rogers uses interchangeably with self. The self-concept is described by Rogers as:

'an organised, configuration of perceptions of the self which are admissible to awareness, it is composed of such elements as the perceptions of one's characteristics and abilities – the concepts of the self in relation to the environment; the value qualities which are perceived as associated with experiences and objects; and the goals and ideals which are perceived as having positive or negative value' (1951, pp. 136–7).

It is during infancy that the human being becomes aware of his or her self and develops a concept or view of that self – the self-concept. The nature of the self-concept, also often referred to as the self-structure, is influenced by interactions with the environment, especially 'significant others' such as parents. In other words, what the infant experiences of the world and how others relate to him or her influence the picture he or she develops of his or her self. Needless to say, the self-concept can develop into a configuration of considerable complexity, given the number of different interactions, messages and situations the growing infant experiences. He or she, when young, will also 'take on' (or internalise) the values of other people as the true version of reality. Many of these messages of course can be contradictory as well as unspoken. The infant is extraordinarily sensitive to subtlety of communication and learns to read body language and facial expression well before verbal language understanding develops.

It is proposed that the self-concept is in a continual process of change throughout our lives and as we encounter an enormous range of situations. This makes us highly complex beings and no wonder it is much easier to think of our self, instead, as a fixed unit. To give an example, it would be much easier to always think of myself as a patient person. However, the reality is that my level of patience varies enormously according to the situation – what I am required to be patient with, my mood, general stress levels, how much sleep I had the night before and a whole host of other factors of which I am probably not aware. This, therefore, makes me cautious about defining myself, or aspects of my self. I can only say how I perceive myself to be in any given moment and I want to be open to the fact that I might perceive myself very differently in another moment. This is not to say that I regard myself as having many selves. Rather, I regard my self as not being a fixed structure, but more of a flexible and ever changing entity.

The idea of values being attached to experiences – i.e. the ability to evaluate positively or negatively our experiences – is another important one. Related to this is the hypothesis of an instinctive, internal valuing process in which human beings, initially as infants, are able to value experiences that serve to satisfy a need. It is the innate tendency to 'know' what is the best direction or optimal experience in pursuit of our maintenance or enhancement. This process Rogers calls the 'organismic valuing process'. It is an ongoing, self-regulating process of evaluating experiences. For example, the infant knows when it is hungry and that this experience is unpleasant. It knows how to communicate its need to be fed and thereby achieve maintenance of this basic biological need. Under the influence of the actualising tendency, this process is occurring from birth and before the development of the self-concept. It is unconscious and instinctive.

However, in Rogers' theory there is one vital need that can dominate everything. This is the need for 'positive regard' or love. As infants, positive regard comes from parents or other significant caregivers. This need for positive regard is, according to Rogers, powerful and overwhelming. We perceive (perception being our reality) that our survival depends upon receiving positive regard, which means that those from whom we most need it have enormous influence on us.

Now this is fine when we are loved and accepted, and *experience* that love and acceptance because it has been communicated effectively, no matter what we do or how we behave, i.e. *unconditionally*. However, readily communicated unconditional positive regard is usually impossible to achieve in practice given, for example, the complexities of our lives and personalities, and our many agendas and responsibilities. The reality is that certain behaviours of the infant invariably attract more approval than others, although rightly so when certain behaviours need to be sanctioned for reasons of safety or social acceptability. Loving and acceptant attitudes, or withholding of love and affection are often, therefore, expressed *on condition* of certain ways of behaving. An obvious example would be a young girl who learns that her Mum will be pleased if she eats everything put on her plate. What is happening, is that from a young age she is acquiring what is termed 'conditions of worth'. We learn that we experience a sense of worth and love when certain conditions are met. Positive regard (worth) is communicated to the girl if everything on her plate gets eaten. The condition of worth here is 'I will love you if you eat everything on your plate', although not necessarily stated in these terms. These conditions (also known as introjected values) can become attached not just to what we do (how we behave), but also to what we think or feel. For example, a boy might learn very readily that if he experiences and shows the powerful emotion of fear when he goes to see the nurse for an injection, his Dad will become impatient and cross with him. If this is the case, the condition of worth is 'I will love you as long as you are not afraid of injections'. Likewise, it could be 'I will love you if you do not make a fuss and always put a brave face on things'.

What we will tend to do, then, is learn to behave in ways to ensure that we receive positive regard, or at least, avoid it being withheld or receiving negative judgements. Furthermore, because the need for positive regard or love is so powerful, we will do whatever we can to receive it, even if it means overriding our internal (organismic) valuing process. Even if the young girl instinctively dislikes the food put on her plate, or perhaps sees harmful mould on the food, she may override this to receive her Mum's approval. In the other example, the boy may learn not to show that he is scared and override his natural, instinctive fear to avoid his Dad's displeasure.

We go on acquiring conditions of worth throughout our lives, for example every time we receive the message 'I like/hate it when you ...', or more powerfully, 'I love/hate you when you ...'. Those conditions acquired in our earliest years will have a particularly powerful influence. They seem to lay down strong templates. Life then offers opportunities and experiences that either reinforce the original templates or create new ones.

I find it interesting, although also disturbing, to reflect upon those conditions of worth that patients may acquire through their experiences of the psychiatric system and encounters with mental health professionals, such as a patient being approved of because he or she is engaging with the help offered (or complying with treatment) and the 'difficult/awkward patient' who is so labelled because of seeming not to want to 'get better'. I will say more about this in Chapter 8.

It is also hypothesised that we have a need for 'positive self-regard'. This is the view we form of ourselves regarding what we think is worthy and good. The development of this, it is postulated, depends upon the messages (and conditions) of worth we first receive from others. How we come to value ourselves depends upon the values we take on from others. High levels of positive self-regard are the consequence of receiving high levels of unconditional positive regard from others. Likewise, lack of positive self-regard is the result of experiencing low levels of positive regard from others. Another way of putting this is that lack of positive regard from others leads to low self-esteem or poor self-regard. Fortunately, where self-esteem is poor from a young age it can be developed later in life, but this will still depend upon being in an affirming, accepting relationship or environment and receiving unconditional positive regard.

Self-regard also includes the ability to evaluate for ourselves what we are experiencing. It is being our own judge. This is necessary in order to become less dependent on others. As part of healthy development towards adulthood and a healthy degree of independence it is important to be able to value our own experiences independently of the evaluations of others. However, such internal valuing will only develop after a process of relying on the values of significant others.

The term Rogers uses to describe this valuing process is 'locus of evaluation'. This is described as *internal* if we rely on our own judgements and trust our own opinions and experience, whilst an *external* locus of evaluation refers to relying on the judgements and values of others. When it comes to evaluations of the self – how we should behave, think or feel in order to receive the other's approval – we are responding to conditions of worth and demonstrating an external locus of evaluation.

Returning to the self-concept then, a significant portion of it will be comprised of conditions of worth, powerfully informing our attitudes and values and especially the view we come to hold of ourselves. It is important not to forget that, as well as parents and significant others, there will also be cultural influences on the developing self-concept. Our culture imposes powerful conditions of worth. Two examples would be our society's current preoccupations with physical appearance and material values, both with strong messages communicated via the media and advertising. The message regularly given is that we are most worthy if we are slim, beautiful and wealthy. It is important also to be aware of the powerful influence of language and how easily the words we use can convey ideas as though they were truths.

A final process to consider in Rogers' hypothesis of personality development is that of 'self-actualisation', which is not the same as that described by Maslow. In Maslow's theory, self-actualisation is the highest level of the so-called 'hierarchy of needs'. It is the fulfilment of all that person's potential and the development of all their unique capacities, at a higher level than meeting more basic human needs such as hunger and physical nurture.

In contrast, Rogers thinks of the process of self-actualisation, specifically, as one of maintaining and enhancing the self-concept. The need to preserve the self-concept is an important one and the individual is engaged in this process even if it causes tension with the overall actualising tendency. The self-actualising tendency can be thought of as a 'subsystem' of the actualising tendency. When these two processes come into conflict this causes psychological disturbance. This is the subject I shall move on to in the next section.

Having outlined Rogers' theory of personality development, I want to add, finally, that I do not see any basic conflict between his ideas and the requirement of a normal biological development of brain structures and functions both pre- and post-natally. Although Rogers' ideas concentrate on 'nurture' and describe largely an 'interpersonal theory' of development, he does not reject the role of 'nature'. It is not a case of either/or, or how much of one and how much of the other that contributes to personality development. Both matter. It has even been suggested that 'in the light of recent research, the "nature or nurture" debate seems to be redundant' (Embleton-Tudor *et al*, 2004, p. 98).

Psychological disturbance: a person-centred view

One misconception of the person-centred approach is that it fails to account fully for psychopathology. Whilst there may be a tendency amongst many person-centred therapists to avoid using such a medical term as psychopathology, there is certainly no denial in the person-centred approach of the reality of psychological disturbance (*see* Chapter 4). What it is not though, is a theory of disease in the sense of describing biological abnormalities.

Crucial to Rogers' understanding of psychological disturbance (or personality disturbance as it is often referred to), is an understanding of the actualising tendency, the self-concept, self-actualisation, and psychological mechanisms of defence. The theory proposed is a generic one and the term Rogers generally uses to explain disturbance is 'incongruence'. Incongruence, like its opposite, congruence, is a term that unfortunately often causes confusion. This is partly, I think, because it is such a general term and has been described in a number of ways. I am grateful here to McMillan (2004) for articulating clearly the two aspects of congruence that are described. The terms he uses to distinguish between these two aspects are *intra*personal and *inter*personal congruence and incongruence. Chapter 8 will consider interpersonal congruence and incongruence, which comprise the communicative aspect that flows from the inner (intrapersonal) state of congruence and incongruence. I am concerned in this section with intrapersonal incongruence – a disturbance *within* individuals.

A variety of other terms have been used interchangeably with incongruence. Terms such as anxiety, inner tension, conflict or discrepancy have been used. I also note two different, but related, ways in which incongruence is said to arise within the individual, or rather, two different ways it is described. First, incongruence can describe the conflict between the actualising tendency and the self-actualising tendency. A good illustration of this can be demonstrated in the story, and film, of 'Billy Elliot', in which Billy's actualising tendency includes the desire and drive to become a ballet dancer. This conflicts with conditions of worth (imposed mainly by his father and brother), which leads to a self-concept that views boys doing ballet as 'sissy'. Instead, he should be learning how to box as the way to becoming a true man in the eyes of his father, brother and culture. Happily the story ends positively because Billy's actualising tendency wins through, despite initial conflicts with his self-concept and self-actualising tendency. He receives enough encouragement and affirmation from his ballet instructor that his self-concept is able to change, which, coupled with the chang-ing attitudes of his father, leads to reduction of inner tension (incongruence). This facilitates the tendency to actualise towards the fulfilment of his desires and dream of becoming a ballet dancer.

The second situation concerns incongruence between the experience of the organism (experience being all that is going on in the organism) and the self-concept. (Instead of using the rather unwieldy term 'organismic experiencing', it would be tempting to use terms such as the 'real self' or 'true self' to describe the experience within the organism. However, this would be misleading since the self-concept is every bit as real or true.) I have already described how the conditions of worth can become incorporated into the self-concept. What follows is an example that aims to demonstrate how aspects of the self-concept can be quite alien to organismic experience, how this results in disturbance, and the mechanisms of defence that are deployed when the self-concept comes under threat. This example also shows again the conflict between the actualising tend-ency of the whole organism and the self-actualising tendency.

A young girl might think she should learn how to cook like her older sisters, and might believe that, like them, she should be good at cooking because this skill seems to run in the family. These ideas form part of her self-concept and have been acquired through receiving conditions of worth from her parents, communicating how much she will be valued and how proud they will be if she continues the family profession of catering. However, she also loves to play the piano (her organismic experience) and her creative tendencies would actually find more natural expression through making music rather than making cakes. Therefore, the actualising tendency that works towards fulfilling her musical potential is in conflict with the self-actualising tendency that is working towards maintaining her self-concept and her belief that becoming a top chef is of much higher status and would earn her greater parental approval than becoming a professional pianist. There is now conflict, or incongruence, between the girl's musical interests and desires and her self-concept that demands she abandon music in favour of developing her cooking skills. In this situation then, she will experience emotional discomfort or some degree of psychological tension. Rogers often refers to this basic discomfort in general terms as anxiety, although recognising that this would express itself in its own unique way according to the degree of incongruence, other features of the personality, and the environmental context. What is meant by environmental context is the freedom the girl has to allow her emotional discomfort into her conscious awareness and give it expression. For example, how permissible would it be for her to acknowledge to her parents her disappointment, or even anger, at not being allowed to con-tinue her piano lessons? How OK is it to own and express anger in the family home? Maybe she has learned from an early age that experiencing anger is taboo, along with challenging parental wishes. Factors such as these will probably influence what psychological defences come into play and the form of expression of psychological distress.

Rogers' concept of psychological defence mechanisms is actually in line with psychoanalytical ideas, although it is a much-simplified version of them in terms of theoretical constructs. Defences are thought of as unconscious psychological processes that enable a person to deal with the threat to the ego (in Freudian terms) or the self-concept in Rogers' terms. Where hypotheses differ is in the nature and origins of psychological conflict and the categorisation of defence mechanisms. In psychoanalysis, numerous types of mechanisms have been postulated such as 'repression', 'projection', 'intellectualisation', 'reaction formation', 'splitting', to name just a few. Rogers, however, describes only two types of defence process. These are 'denial' and 'distortion'. He seems not to be interested in the variety of complex theories of Freud and his followers, presumably partly in keeping with his desire not to define, label or overly explain psychological mechanisms. Distortion can be viewed as a form of denial (partial denial) depending on how strong the defence needs to be or the type of experience that needs to be defended against.

In order to understand how defence mechanisms come into play it is important to understand that, according to Rogers, the self-concept concerns experience available to a person's conscious awareness. Defences are deployed to keep material out of a person's conscious awareness, or in other words, when the integrity of the self-concept is under threat. Threatening experiences are those which don't fit with the self-concept and which would be in conflict with the self-concept were they to be accurately perceived or 'symbolised'. (Rogers uses the terms 'awareness', 'symbolisation' and 'consciousness' interchangeably.) Threatening experiences may therefore be 're-interpreted' in the defence process to become less threatening, or less in conflict with the self-concept. The tendency to self-actualise (to actualise and maintain the self-concept) can be very powerful, whatever the self-concept.

This process can be illustrated by returning to the earlier example. Should the girl's younger brother take up playing the piano and be encouraged by their parents to become a professional musician, her natural emotional responses might be intense jealousy and anger. However, she has also come to think of herself as someone who maintains a calm and gentle manner at all times and has come to believe that anger is a negative and unhelpful emotion. These ideas and beliefs are part of her self-concept as a result of conditions of worth from her parents ('I will love you if you are gentle' or 'I disapprove when you are angry'). Feeling and expressing anger towards her brother will not, therefore, fit with her view of herself and how she should behave, so it is denied from her awareness. She may not be at all conscious of her anger. A distortion, or partial symbolisation, of emotional experience would occur were she to allow herself some feelings of irritation whenever her brother is practising the piano. However, she might claim that this is due to his getting the notes wrong and it sounding unpleasant. The experience of anger is distorted into seemingly rational and justifiable irritation.

Further examples of defence mechanisms are as follows:

- A man believes that he should not experience or show fear in the face of danger. Should he then find himself in a frightening situation in which his pulse rate rises and he becomes sweaty, he might misinterpret these normal physiological reactions to fear by believing he has a physical condition that caused this. An example of denial of fear.

- A woman who is unable to contemplate the prospect of losing a tennis game, due to a strong need to always be the best at whatever she does, might make all sorts of excuses as to why she lost, none of them relating to her performance. An example of denial (of the reason she lost, if due to being beaten by a better player).
- Believing that I am no good at something might lead me to conclude that doing well in it must be the result of good luck rather than ability. An example of distortion.
- Patients who believe that they are not worthy of receiving help are likely to misinterpret the care shown to them by a nurse or doctor as that person not really caring but just doing their job. In other words, they believe that the caring attitude cannot possibly be genuine. (When patients voice this to me I occasionally reply that it is because I care that I do this job and not the other way around, although the strength of their defence may prevent them from believing me.) An example of denial of the reason for care.
- Psychotic symptoms such as delusional beliefs could be regarded as a denial or distortion of reality.

Many of the above examples actually demonstrate that often there isn't a clear and easy distinction between denial and distortion because of the complexity of our experiences and interweaving of many thoughts and feelings (and defensive processes) in any given situation.

It is important to note that 'good' experiences as well as 'bad' ones will be denied or distorted if they do not fit with the self-concept. In fact, this is a barrier for many people I see recovering from mental distress/illness. Many patients who come to the attention of psychiatric services have a pre-existing low sense of self-worth and because of this believe that they simply do not deserve to feel good about themselves, feel well or 'get better'. Their self-concept may, in extreme cases, include the belief that they deserve to be ill or feel wretched about themselves. In this instance, admitting to self-awareness the emergence of good, positive feelings will be very threatening as it does not fit with the self-concept of deserving to feel bad. Recovery will therefore often be a long process of movements both forward and backward. I think this is a very commonly overlooked issue amongst mental health professionals all too keen to point out to a patient that they look better and that there seem to be signs of improvement that deserve celebration. Mental health and a feeling of well-being are not the desired goal for everyone, and for people with self-concepts full of self-loathing they may be a frightening prospect.

Finally in this section, I want to briefly consider the person-centred approach to psychopathology in terms of the categories of mental disturbance psychiatry traditionally uses. Person-centred theory here remains very general. Essentially the different forms of disturbance or types of illnesses, as classified in psychiatry, are viewed as different ways of experiencing and expressing incongruence. These different forms will depend upon a host of factors such as personality, biochemistry, genetic predisposition, the nature and degree of inner conflict or threat (incongruence) and environment. Thus the 'biopsychosocial model' of psychiatry, which tries to view mental disturbance holistically, can, in my opinion, be considered along with Rogers' theory of personality disturbance.

Rogers' theory of what occurs in severe mental disturbance such as psychosis is simply that defences have been overwhelmed. They have failed to keep experiences out of awareness. The personality therefore becomes 'disorganised' and perceptions of reality become considerably altered. This will inevitably result in disturbances of thinking, emotions, perceptions and behaviour.

Some criticisms of Rogers' theory of personality and behaviour

One of the criticisms sometimes made of the person-centred approach is that it lacks a theory of personality. I hope that I have demonstrated otherwise in this chapter. If the criticism is that Rogers' theory is fairly rudimentary when it comes to the development of types of psychopathology, and that 'it provides very little help in understanding the wide varieties of disturbing and pathological experiences and behaviours . . .' (Cain, 1993, p. 135–136), then I agree. Rogers is less interested in providing explanatory mechanisms. However, for me this would not count as a criticism. Cain would clearly regard it as one of the inadequacies of a person-centred theory of disturbance that, for example, there is lacking a comprehensive account of the development of neurosis, as opposed to psychosis. I imagine many mental health professionals would be similarly frustrated not to have a comprehensive explanatory theory that also, perhaps, takes full account of biological factors. For Rogers though, a detailed understanding of the cause of psychological disturbance, i.e. the cause of incongruence, is relatively unimportant. This is because, as a therapist, he would aim to behave towards disturbed and distressed individuals in the same way whatever the cause, and however complex the disturbance. Nevertheless, most mental health professionals do not practise as therapists, and in mental health services there is a clear requirement for assessment leading to diagnosis and then treatment, for which the issue of causality (or aetiology) is important.

The other criticism of person-centred personality theory I want to acknowledge, although refute, is that it takes an overly positive view of human nature and lacks an account of evil, leading frequently to the charge that person-centred practitioners are naïve and misguided. Rogers does indeed view the basic nature of human beings as constructive and not destructive. Another word he often uses to describe the basic nature of persons is 'trustworthy'. Unfortunately, the important part of the equation Rogers also stresses, is often ignored or overlooked by his critics. This is the *necessity of certain conditions* for this constructive potential (the tendency to actualise) to manifest itself. Rogers does not, therefore, disregard the reality of evil. He sees clearly that all human beings have the capacity to behave in evil, cruel and destructive ways. He states:

> 'I do not have a Pollyanna view of human nature. I am quite aware that out of defensiveness and inner fear individuals can and do behave in ways which are horribly destructive, immature, regressive, antisocial, hurtful' (1995/1956, p. 21).

However, he sees such behaviour as depending on social conditioning and cultural influences. (There is much in keeping here with behaviourism.) Rogers also regards voluntary choice as having a crucial part to play, although this raises difficult questions as to what influences choice. In summary then, Rogers sees behaviours, rather than people, as evil.

This clearly contrasts with the views of other prominent psychologists who believe that there is an evil impulse within human nature. Freud's view is that we have inherent aggressive instincts within the unconscious and that these lead us to behave destructively. This continues to be the view of many in the psychoanalytical world who would see human nature as needing to be tamed and controlled. Likewise, many theologians and Christians would view Rogers' ideas regarding the basic trustworthiness of human nature as naïve and quite simply wrong for not taking account of notions of 'Original Sin' or evil and demonic forces in the universe.

Thorne (2003) does point out though, that 'Rogers was not wholly satisfied with his own arguments in favour of man's essential trustworthiness despite the almost overwhelming positive data from his therapeutic experience' (p. 84). In other words, despite his extensive experience as a therapist and in serious thinking and debate with prominent psychologists and theologians of the day, he does acknowledge that his understanding of and answer to the question of evil were not complete. Fortunately, others have taken up this debate such as Thorne (1991, 1998) and Worsley (2005).

The 'fully functioning person'

The 'fully functioning person' is another of Rogers' key concepts. A brief consideration of it here completes this exploration of his theory of personality and behaviour. Essentially, the concept describes a person engaged in a set of processes – of 'becoming' – rather than in a fixed state. It also represents an ideal. The fully functional person is a hypothetical person.

Rogers describes the characteristics of the fully functioning person in his 1959 paper and comprehensive theory statement. Merry (1999, p. 40) helpfully summarises these characteristics in simple terms.

'The fully functioning person would:

Be open to experience.
Exhibit no defensiveness.
Be able to interpret experience accurately.
Have a flexible rather than static self-concept open to change through experience.
Trust in his or her own experiencing process and develop values in accordance with that experience.
Have no conditions of worth and experience unconditional self-regard.
Be able to respond to new experiences openly.
Be guided by his or her own valuing process through being fully aware of all experience, without the need for denial or distortion of any of it.
Be open to feedback from his or her environment and make realistic changes resulting from that feedback.
Live in harmony with others and experience the rewards of mutual positive regard.'

Essentially, the fully functioning person is completely congruent and integrated. Such a person, Rogers believes, is able to embrace 'existential living'. By this he means they are able to live fully in the here and now with personal inner freedom, with all its accompanying exciting, creative, but also challenging, aspects. The theory and practice of the person-centred approach is to facilitate the development of such a person. That this is possible is borne out by Rogers' experience of offering a particular relationship and facilitative environment. Worthy of note, however, is the view of Embleton-Tudor *et al*, who 'prefer to think that the organism is always functioning as fully as it possibly can given the conditions within it and around it' (2004, p. 48).

On a final note, I recently read 'Going Sane', a recently published book by Adam Phillips (2005), a psychoanalyst and writer. In this book he explores the concept of sanity, believing that whilst people are fascinated by madness 'there has been no particular enthusiasm for the idea of sanity' (p. 6). He states also that 'there are no accounts of what a sane life would look like' (p. 9) and he attempts to provide a contemporary account of sanity. It is a shame that he does not refer to Rogers' concept of the fully functioning person. Clearly it is not the case that no one has attempted to tease out and explore characteristics of a psychologically healthy and adjusted person, even if the word sanity is not one Rogers uses. In Phillips' attempt to provide an account of sanity, he appears to have read neither Rogers' concepts of the fully functioning person nor Rogers' description of the 'Person of Tomorrow' (1980).

References

Bozarth J (1998) *Person-Centred Therapy: A Revolutionary Paradigm*. PCCS Books, Ross-on-Wye.

Cain DJ (1993) The uncertain future of client-centred counselling. *Journal of Humanistic Education and Development*, **31**: 133–139.

Embleton-Tudor L, Keemar K, Tudor K, Valentine J and Worrall M (2004) *The Person-Centred Approach: A Contemporary Introduction*. Palgrave Macmillan, Basingstoke.

Hjelle L and Ziegler D (1992) *Personality Theories: Basic Assumptions, Research and Applications*. McGraw-Hill, New York.

McMillan M (2004) *The Person-Centred Approach to Therapeutic Change*. Sage publications, London.

Merry T (1999) *Learning and Being in Person-Centred Counselling* (2nd edition). PCCS Books, Ross-on-Wye.

Phillips A (2005) *Going Sane*. Hamish Hamilton, London.

Rogers C (1951) *Client-Centred Therapy: Its Current Practice, Implications And Theory*. Constable, London.

Rogers C (1959) A theory of therapy, personality, and interpersonal relationships, as developed in the client-centred framework. In S Koch (ed) *Psychology: a study of a science*. Study 1. Volume 3. *Formulations of the person and the social context*. McGraw-Hill, New York, pp. 184–256.

Rogers C (1980) *A Way of Being*. Houghton Mifflin, Boston, MA.

Rogers C (1990) Client-Centred Therapy. In H Kirschenbaum and V Henderson (eds) *Carl Rogers: Dialogues*. Constable, London, pp. 9–38. (Original work published 1959)

Rogers C (1995) What Understanding and Acceptance Mean to Me. *Journal of Humanistic Psychology*, **35(4)**: 7–22. (Transcript of a talk delivered in 1956)

Schmid P (1998) 'On Becoming a *Person*-Centred Approach': A Person-Centred Understanding of the Person. In B Thorne and E Lambers (eds) *Person-Centred Therapy. A European Perspective*. Sage publications, London, pp. 38–52.

Thorne B (1991) *Person-Centred Counselling. Therapeutic and Spiritual Dimensions*. Whurr Publishers, London.

Thorne B (1998) *Person-centred Counselling and Christian Spirituality. The Secular and the Holy*. Whurr Publishers, London.

Thorne B (2003) *Carl Rogers*. Sage publications, London.

Tudor K and Worrall M (2006) *Person-Centred Therapy. A Clinical Philosophy*. Routledge, London.

Wilkins P (2003) *Person-Centred Therapy in Focus*. Sage Publications, London.

Worsley R (2005) The Concept of Evil as a Key to the Therapist's Use of the Self. In S Joseph and R Worsley (eds) *Person-Centred Psychopathology. A Positive Psychology of Mental Health*. PCCS Books, Ross-on-Wye, pp. 146–157.

Further reading

- Rogers' earliest formulation of personality theory is contained in the form of 19 propositions in one of his most well known books *Client-Centred Therapy: Its Current Practice, Implications and Theory* (1951). Constable.
- *Person-Centred Therapy in Focus* (2003) by Paul Wilkins (Sage) provides a scholarly exploration and refutation of some of the main criticisms of the person-centred approach, such as it being naïve, sentimental and not scientifically rigorous.
- One recent development of person-centred personality theory is the concept 'configurations of self', explored in *Person-Centred Therapy Today: New Frontiers in Theory and Practice* (2000) by Dave Mearns and Brian Thorne (Sage).
- An advanced understanding of person-centred theory is presented in *Person-Centred Therapy. A Clinical Philosophy* (2006) by Keith Tudor and Mike Worrall (Routledge).

Chapter 3

Who has the power and where is the expertise?

'Our deepest fear is not that we are inadequate. Our deepest fear is that we are powerful beyond measure.'

From Nelson Mandela's Inaugural speech, 1994

Introduction

In recent years the issues of power, control and authority have featured heavily in the rhetoric of government health policy and its programme of service reform. 'Patient empowerment', 'partnership' and the need to challenge 'medical paternalism' are often discussed these days. 'Shifting the balance of power' (2001) is the title of a Department of Health document which outlines an initiative intending to give more power and control over budgets to patients and staff on the front line. Issues of power and control are increasingly under the spotlight in many areas of health care services, particularly their organisation and delivery. We have also entered an era in which the concept of authority is questioned and its role challenged. The focus of this chapter is the complex and challenging issue of power and the related subject of expertise, since these are issues in which the person-centred approach adopts a clear and radical stance. In fact, these issues lie at the very heart of this approach.

Politicians, managers and policy-makers try to address concepts of power by, for example, responding to the requests of patients and user-groups for more influence and power in the way mental health services are organised. This would, you would think, warm the hearts of enthusiasts of the person-centred approach. Unfortunately, reality does not match the rhetoric. In fact, it often demonstrates contemptible hypocrisy, since the political and managerial agenda is to retain firm control over the nature of clinical practice and how services are structured, delivered and funded. Therefore, anyone working in the NHS, particularly in mental health settings, who takes seriously the issue of power and the ethical dimensions surrounding it, is likely to experience considerable tension, frustration and dismay. It is the issues of power and expertise that cause me some of my most profound personal and professional conflicts and dilemmas. Quite simply, my own theoretical and philosophical position, generally in keeping with that of the person-centred approach, feels out of step with the organisational context in which I work. I often experience my personal ethics and values being compromised, and in extreme cases my integrity seriously challenged, possibly even violated by the way the organisation requires me to work.

Teasing out some of these conflicts and attempting to shed brighter light on them has also revealed my own feelings of ambivalence around power and expertise.

41

This chapter has therefore been a particular struggle to write. In wrestling with these areas I suspect I am not alone with my difficulties as a mental health professional seeking to be reflective and sensitive to the complex dynamics of power. The more a person tries to be person-centred, the more the issue of power will be fundamental to clinical practice. It is questionable whether it is even possible to practise the person-centred approach within a mental health setting in its purest form, i.e., faithfully adhering to Rogers' original theory. It may well be that this fundamental clash of theory, philosophy and practice regarding the issue of power, between the person-centred approach and traditional psychiatric practice, is the reason it is so rare to find person-centred psychologists, counsellors or psychotherapists working in mental health services. Person-centred practitioners are likely to view much of psychiatric practice as fundamentally disempowering of patients and working within mental health services may present too many conflicts with and compromises of their approach.

In what follows, I aim to introduce some concepts of power and expertise as they relate to health care contexts, the practice of psychiatry and mental health services. I intend to acknowledge those instances where the issue of power, because of its potential for abuse, is a cause for serious thinking and reflection. However, I also want to 'rescue' the concept of power from its mostly negative associations. It is also possible for power to be seen in terms of its positive and constructive potential. In fact, there is nothing negative in some of the ways in which it is defined. Power has been described as, for example, 'the ability to do or act'; 'influence, or authority'; 'an influential person, group, or organisation'; 'vigour, energy'; 'an active property or function' (Oxford English Reference Dictionary, 1996).

Finally, I shall introduce person-centred theory and understanding as it relates to power and expertise.

Thinking about power

When discussing mental health services and the practice of psychiatry, the word and concept of 'power' will often evoke negative and uncomfortable feelings. Power tends to be associated with concepts of control, abuse, coercion and authority. It is not hard to find academic literature of a critical nature. Examples include the historian and philosopher Michel Foucault's examination of madness in 'Madness and Civilisation' (1977), and Ivan Illich's discussion of the damaging effects of medicalisation and other harmful processes of the health care system in 'Limits to Medicine' (1995). More for the lay person, Tana Dineen (1999) looks at the so-called 'Psychology Industry' and explores how people are turned into 'victims'. This is a view shared by Lucy Johnstone, a psychologist, whose book 'Users and Abusers of Psychiatry. A Critical Look at Traditional Psychiatric Practice' (2000) provides a powerful critique of the whole psychiatric system. The experiences of service-users and carers also make themselves increasingly known through the development of organised protest groups and activist networks. Much writing by people who refer to themselves as 'survivors', includes accounts of their experiences of being oppressed by psychiatry.

The psychiatric institution is a powerful one. Examples abound throughout the history of psychiatry where power has been misused and abused, from the days of the Victorian asylum to Nazi programmes of euthanasia of the mentally ill, to recent times when Soviet political dissidents were wrongly diagnosed with metal illness (described as having delusions of reform) and admitted to mental institutions. This latter example is as recent as the 1970s and '80s. The use of psychiatry for social control has been a dominating theme in its history and gave impetus to the anti-psychiatry movement in the 1960s. Unfortunately, as I shall discuss later, the issue of social control is not confined to the past.

Authoritarian power within psychiatry

To begin with, psychiatry is powerful in the way it influences thinking about the causes and management of mental disorder, in determining the dominant language of 'illness' and scientific discourse and in the way it struggles to respect or tolerate alternative viewpoints.

In the context of relationship, it is the *balance* of power that is the focus of attention. Natiello (2001) describes the concept of 'authoritarian power' or 'power-over', in which 'the practice of power is often grounded in the belief that power is a coercive force that we exercise over the earth and over one another' (p. 60). In other words, one party has more power than the other and is in a greater position, therefore, of control, authority and influence.

Within the mental health system it is the concept of 'authoritarian power' that seems to receive the most attention, much of it highly critical, particularly from those with the least power. The exercise of power in psychiatric practice certainly does, I believe, deserve close scrutiny and reform in many areas. For example, serious thinking about the structures in which care is provided is urgently needed. Coercion to comply with treatment in psychiatric hospitals and in community mental health care is alive and well.

One obvious reason for the need for vigorous challenge of the use of authoritarian power is that much psychological distress springs from a feeling of powerlessness. Abuse, socio-economic deprivation and emotional neglect are well-documented contributors to mental distress and illness and all are in some way associated with powerlessness. Mental distress itself can take the form of diminished functioning or loss of freedom, i.e. a loss of power. Coming into contact with a powerful institution such as a psychiatric service, whose way of working is often to exercise 'power-over', is likely to further increase a person's distress, psychological disturbance and feelings of powerlessness. Therefore, as Proctor says, 'the way to deal with difficulties that stem from abuse, deprivation and powerlessness is not to impose further power and control through the psychiatric system' (2002, p. 4).

There are many ways in which psychiatry can exercise authoritarian power. What follows is a brief outline of some of the more obvious areas where 'power over' patients can occur. (This is not to mention extreme cases of abuse such as the exploitation of role and position for financial, emotional or sexual gain, in which patients are singled out because they are vulnerable and lack the power to resist. It is likely that many of these abusers are attracted to working with mentally vulnerable people precisely because it enhances their own fragile sense of power and sense of being in control.)

To begin with it is sometimes argued that the word 'patient' itself represents a power imbalance, with patients passively receiving care from experts. It is for this reason that the terms 'client' or 'service-user' are often preferred in mental health settings, although the traditional 'patient' label seems to have been retained in other areas of health care so far. The problem with this argument is that whilst the health professional is in a powerful position, an assumption is being made about the patient's relative lack of power and passivity which may not be the case. Neither do I believe, as some do, that when there is a power imbalance, particularly in the context of health care, it is intrinsically oppressive.

The 'medical model', the predominant model in psychiatry (of which more will be said in Chapters 5 and 6), involves a power imbalance in the relationship between professional and patient. Expert knowledge, with its corresponding technical medical language, is utilised in the processes of assessment, diagnosis and deciding on treatment, usually according to a scientific, objective under-standing of the problem. Many patients object to the medical model for its paternalistic style of interaction and relationship, particularly when the profes-sional is authoritarian in his or her manner and is not particularly interested in hearing the views of the patient. These are genuine problems. However, in defence of many practitioners working in this way, it is not necessarily based on the desire to control the patient. Often it is based primarily on simple faith in the scientific paradigm, although this is not to say that this faith should not be challenged, particularly concerning mental illness. Another contributing factor in the use of the medical model is simply the fact that it usually makes fewer demands on time and energy. The medical model is time efficient, and often mentally less taxing. Given the pressures on mental health services and on professionals, taking time to listen to patients' views or explore alternative (non-scientific) ways of understanding problems, is often put aside in order to get through the volume of people referred to services. Many lines of argument can be pursued both for and against the use of the medical model, particularly within psychiatry. The disease model of mental illness (sometimes referred to as the biomedical model) that views illness as having an underlying physical cause, can also be disempowering for many patients. More will be said about the disease model in Chapter 4.

In psychiatry, probably the most obvious area in which issues of power and authority receive critical attention is when patients are detained in hospital and treated against their will under mental health legislation. This power of certain mental health professionals, sanctioned by law, can instil enormous fear and anger in people on the receiving end, the psychological consequences of which can be experienced long-term. Whether these powers are appropriate and justified should regularly be a subject for ethical and philosophical debate. Unfortunately, the lack of debate can be the result of lack of time and space for mental health professionals in which to think critically, debate and reflect.

It is also important to acknowledge that what the current government and much of society seem to want, is to eradicate the risk of the occasional and un-predictable tragedy when violence, particularly homicide, is committed by some-one with a mental illness. This is despite the fact that people with mental illness are much more likely to commit suicide (Appleby, 1992), and the fact that by far the majority of cases of homicide are committed by people who do not have a mental illness (Taylor and Gunn, 1999). Szmukler (2000) has highlighted the tendency to exaggerate the link between mental illness and dangerous behaviour.

The current government has a strong public protection agenda. The attitude within society towards risk and towards people with mental illness (stoked up by the media) has had profound consequences on psychiatric practice. There continues to be an increase in the number of people detained in hospital against their will, with an increase of compulsory admissions in England by 63% between 1984 and 1996 (Hotopf, Wall *et al*, 2000). This is partly due to mental health professionals' fear of being blamed if disaster were to occur. Many psychiatrists and mental health social workers feel as though they have become so-called 'agents of social control' and that they are being asked to implement the authoritarian and controlling agenda of the government, as well as pandering to society's fears. Could this in fact be an exploitation and abuse of the psychiatric profession and other mental health professionals by the government and sections of the public? This situation would certainly have worsened had the government's recent proposals for reform of the mental health act been implemented (Thornicroft and Szmukler, 2005). Under the recently proposed parliamentary bill, now dropped, authoritarian power could have been exercised to detain indefinitely people (to whom the government have given the diagnostic label 'dangerous severe personality disorder') who might present a risk to the public, even when they have not committed an offence. In short, psychiatrists would have been able and expected to use more often, powers to detain people. We would have been required even more to consider public safety issues before therapeutic concerns. Szmukler and Holloway powerfully describe the proposals as 'the iron hand of coercion fitted within the velvet glove of legalism and expressed in a rhetoric of care' (2000a, p. 14) and that using mental health legislation to protect others and reduce risk will increase the scope for abuse (2000b). Unfortunately, amendments to the existing bill may yet lead to abuses of power and coercion because the government are still intent on implementing its public protection agenda.

Prescribing medication is another area in which there is much potential for control and coercion. 'Is the patient complying with medication?' could easily be interpreted as 'Is the patient doing as they are told and adhering to the treatment plan?' The term 'compliance' describes a patient's behaviour and mental health professionals' concern that a patient is cooperating with treatment. This can often indicate a lack of genuine respect for patient autonomy. The assumption is made by mental health professionals that they know what is best for the patient. However, there have been efforts in recent years, reflecting the changes in health care culture generally, to think differently about how patients take medication. This change is evident by increasing use of new terminology. The 'Medicine Partnership', an organisation created by the Department of Health in 2002, is trying to replace the concept of compliance with that of 'concordance'. Concordance is concerned with the process of consultation and a shared approach to making decisions when it comes to the issue of medication. Within the consultation patients are supposed to be given sufficient information to help make decisions. Or should it be to help make the 'right' decision? Heath (2003) makes the point that concordance might still be coercion, but in a subtle and more covert way. In other words, education improves compliance, or the more understanding a person has (through being given certain information in a certain way), the more likely they are to co-operate. In psychiatric settings, particularly in in-patient environments, whether a patient is complying with medication is a regular preoccupation of mental health professionals. Is the patient obeying the rules? And if not, how can we persuade patients to 'see sense', to agree with the professionals' point of view? How can we use our power and authority to persuade patients into taking medication are questions we ask ourselves, although not usually quite so explicitly.

Further examples of areas in which there is potential for misuse of authoritarian power are those of 'consent to treatment' and patient confidentiality. 'Informed consent', as it is now often referred to, is an issue that has rightly come under much closer scrutiny in recent years. However, giving patients the right information, in sufficient amounts and in the right way, is a difficult task and one to which not all professionals will be committed and take seriously, and the health professional is still the one who decides what information to impart. Likewise, thoughtless and sloppy approaches towards patient confidentiality are not as rare as they should be. Knowing highly personal details about patients is a powerful position to be in. How often are we mindful of this? What and *how* information about patients is shared, are issues that deserve great sensitivity but which regularly do not receive it.

Professional hierarchies and relationships with colleagues

Amongst professional helpers doctors are often seen as the worst offenders of misusing power or behaving in an authoritarian manner. One of the most common criticisms of doctors is that they are arrogant, which implies an awareness of their status and authority. The medical profession is a powerful one, certainly in the eyes of the public, despite the current government's efforts to erode medical power. Doctors have plenty of opportunity to abuse and misuse their power, with colleagues as much as with patients.

The medical profession, particularly within hospitals, is in my experience often lacking awareness of the dynamics of power, having grown accustomed to its role, method of working, the various power structures within health care environments, and because, throughout medical training, such power and its use are rarely questioned. We seem to accept the status and hierarchies within our profession, knowing our rank and codes of behaviour (e.g. rules of communication) that accompany it. We have learnt to accept medical authority and we often expect this from other professions and patients too. This is the established order of things. It will be a long time before the average junior doctor criticises a consultant's actions without anxiety or fear for the consequences. Likewise, it will be a long time before bullying by senior medical colleagues is readily challenged and exposed.

When popular media psychiatrist Raj Persaud extols in 'Hospital Doctor' (2004, p. 36), a medical newspaper, the virtues of Machiavelli's guide to power, my blood runs cold. He is not encouraging doctors to be ruthless tyrants, but he clearly suggests the value of some of the strategies Machiavelli outlined in his most celebrated work 'The Prince' (1513) – a guide for those seeking to have power over others. Persaud notes such things as 'wearing a mask' and 'making others need you'. It is difficult to know whether he is genuinely encouraging doctors to adopt some of these basic Machiavellian principles as a way of 'acquiring, wielding and (once you've got it) hanging on to power', or whether he is simply highlighting the power-based rules of the medical profession. Certainly when he writes 'the art of gaining power is to make others dependent on you and make yourself independent of them', he fuels the perception in many quarters, including the media and amongst many politicians, that doctors are power-mongers who cannot be trusted, and who need to be controlled. Persaud, for all the good he does in attempting to demystify and de-stigmatise mental illness and educate the public, is nevertheless the powerful and stereotypical expert. He is also the kind of expert whose clear preferences lie in the world of scientific explanations and hard-headed objectivity, rather than subjective experience, meaning and values. It is in the subjective world of meaning and values where issues of power and control are most sensitively appreciated. It is in questioning basic values that we become aware of the potentially destructive aspects of authoritarian power.

Bullying and power-games exist in professions that are competitive and hierarchical in their structure and organisation, such as the medical profession, where titles are badges of status and importance. Medical newspapers and journals regularly report stories of bullying and intimidation of medical students, junior doctors and ethnic minority doctors in particular. 37% of UK junior doctors reported workplace bullying in one survey (Quine, 2002). There still exist medical educators who take a punitive approach to teaching and training and believe, or behave as though they believe, that the way to teach is through instilling fear. Medical soap operas are good at portraying this, albeit often in a deliberately exaggerated way. Thankfully formal medical education is now becoming more enlightened. Nevertheless, doctors' feelings of being exploited and controlled, particularly those whose work is hospital based, are remarkably common and a major contributing factor to a demoralised medical workforce in the UK. Could this also be one of the contributory factors to misuses of power over patients? Bullied doctors have to gain a sense of power from somewhere.

The nursing profession is also hierarchical. 'Matron' (or 'modern matron' to use the new term) and 'sister' are powerful titles and power lies not just in their title. Bullying exists within the nursing profession also. Any profession in which authoritarian power is the dominant paradigm is one that can attract bullies. Unfortunately, in the high-intensity, pressured and target-driven environment of the NHS, bullying will flourish. So will the 'them' and 'us' attitudes that exist between, for example, doctors and nurses and other professional groups where power imbalances exist. Achieving targets and pursuing the more immediate agenda of patient care will always be perceived as more important than taking seriously the power dynamics of professional relationships. Rarely is there the time to reflect on power dynamics within our professional relationships. But neither, it seems to me, is there the inclination.

There is something seriously disturbed and dysfunctional about an organisation that seems to tolerate bullying and aggressive behaviours from ward managers, senior managers, consultants or anyone in a position of power, despite efforts from time to time to raise awareness of this issue. However, perhaps we shouldn't forget the aggressiveness of our political establishments and the power monger-ing that permeates our culture generally.

Organisational power

Power can also be considered more widely in terms of the organisation within which various professions work. The power dynamics within mental health organisations, their general politics, policies and procedures, directly influence psychiatric practice and how people with mental distress and illness are treated.

I have already mentioned how the government's previously proposed mental health legislation would have put the mental health service in a stronger role of social control, in effect giving it more power.

Modern day politics is based on authoritarian power. Power and control cascade down from central government, from politicians to managers to clinicians and front-line workers, and the majority on the front-line often feel powerless to significantly influence policy and management decisions. Radical alternatives to traditional power structures do exist, but they are challenging to implement and risky. They rely on placing more emphasis on relationship, on trust and on collaboration (power sharing), but this would also require a major cultural change. Traditional systems of control of, and within, organisations would be seen as no longer useful or effective, and would therefore be dismantled. What would be required from those in positions of leadership to achieve this, would be a willingness to let go of authoritarian power and control, and this requires great courage, as well as preparedness to tolerate discomfort. It would require leaders to recognise that leadership does not equate with control. Unfortunately, in my observation of institutions and organisations, including mental health services, the common perception of leadership is the ability to influence (often taking the form of manipulation), to persuade and to control. What is not recognised is that 'successful leadership is counterintuitive. It necessitates entrusting others with responsibility' (Harrison and Gray, 2003).

Natiello has written about this so-called *'collaborative power'*, pointing out that 'the tenets of collaborative power are inherent in the theory of the person-centred approach' (2001, p. 62). For her, collaboration is 'full of heart and soul, and even love. It is based on trust, mutuality and respectful relationships between all participants in an organisation' (p. 84). Hirschhorn (1997) describes collaboration within organisations and highlights the need for creating a culture of openness and transparency. The difficulty here of course is being able to tolerate feelings of vulnerability, being honest about uncertainties or mistakes. These qualities are in short supply in most of our leaders and managers of organisations, including the NHS. There seems to be little room for values that place an emphasis on deepening our working relationships, on being responsive to each other and on finding ways to develop co-operation. Hirschhorn also describes being more 'psychologically present' (p. 9), by which he means bringing more of ourselves to the workplace – our ideas, feelings and values. This latter point is emphasised by Natiello who also refers to collaborative leaders needing to be authentic persons.

Collaborative power does not involve doing away with notions of authority. Instead of the authoritarian, power-over model, the concept of 'personal authority' becomes important, built on deepening our relationship with ourselves and with each other. Relationship qualities and attitudes lie at the heart of the person-centred approach, an approach that offers a powerful alternative to the current ethos of organisations in which 'authority is now vested in rules rather than relationships' (Hirschhorn, 1997, p. 58). Likewise, effective leadership does not mean having no authority but understanding and using it differently.

Managing feelings of powerlessness

It is a paradox that for all the power that, as a mental health professional and psychiatrist, I have and I am perceived to have by the public and patients (sometimes including the idea that I can read minds), so often I also feel very powerless. I regularly feel powerless to make a significant and sustained positive impact on many of my patients' mental health. I cannot 'cure' mental illness or remove many of the contributing factors, especially when those factors are rooted in social issues. At best I might be able to minimise distress or temporarily alleviate symptoms. I often feel unable to provide a decent level of care for people in the way I would like because I do not have the resources. I regularly lack time to listen, as well as lack a range of services and individuals to whom I can refer and which would enable me to offer a holistic approach to management and care. I feel powerless to influence policy and shape services, as mentioned earlier. Put all this together and it is tempting to believe that any power I have as a psychiatrist is no more than an illusion. One of the conclusions this leads me to is the vital importance of supervision to manage my feelings of powerlessness. One of the dangers of deep feelings of powerlessness is that it can lead to destructive or punitive behaviour by way of compensation. Supervision helps me to guard against this, and the dangers of embarking on 'power-trips', particularly in situations where I can demonstrate my knowledge and opinions. I need to be alert to when my need for power and control can contaminate the helping relationship. Supervision also enables me to explore and find my own genuine and constructive power within situations that might at first engender feelings of powerlessness. Good supervision should be empowering.

Thinking about expertise and experts

'Psychiatry has created a niche of expertise for itself, as if possessing a special mystique, a unique wisdom and authority', so says Terry Lynch in his book 'Beyond Prozac' (2004, p. 382). He criticises the psychiatric system and the 'expert' professional who tells patients what they need, and fails to hear the patient's view. These sentiments are ones many person-centred practitioners would, I am sure, agree with.

Carl Rogers generally dislikes experts and in many ways the development of the person-centred approach could be viewed as a backlash against the all-knowing and all-powerful experts often to be found, certainly in Rogers' day, within the schools of psychoanalysis and behaviourism. He is scornful of those professionals who use their expertise to hide behind and protect themselves, creating a mystique, and thus enhancing their power over others. For Rogers, it is vital to relate as a person and not as a distant professional. It is likely therefore that, according to Thorne, 'Rogers' ideas threaten those whose professional identity resides chiefly in their psychological knowledge and in their capacity to embody the role of "expert"' (2003, p.66). For such people, being an expert avoids feelings of vulnerability and uncertainty. Rogers' ideas and the person-centred approach will also threaten those who are fearful of relating deeply as persons and who would prefer to keep out their own emotional experiencing from interactions with patients. The person-centred approach will not appeal to mental health professionals whose world of work is predominantly intellectually structured, perhaps partly through fear of being changed or challenged by engaging with the emotional as well as cognitive worlds of patients. But are person-centred criticisms of experts always balanced and fair?

When I was studying for a diploma in person-centred counselling, one of the regular features of my course (and of many person-centred counselling courses) was the 'community meeting'. This was a twice-weekly large group meeting for all trainees and trainers. It was unstructured, with no agenda other than that determined by its participants. It was a meeting in which anything could happen and any topic or issue could be raised for discussion or airing of feelings. I remember on one occasion the topic of being an expert came up and quite an animated discussion ensued. The thrust of the arguments being developed was overwhelmingly negative towards experts, and professional helpers in particular. Several people recounted their personal stories of incidents in which they felt abused by the expert's authoritarian manner. I also remember feeling distinctly uncomfortable as a member of the community who had up until that point invested years of training to become a doctor (a medical expert) and further developed some expertise whilst training to be a psychiatrist. I did not feel personally attacked, but I did feel indirectly condemned for being an expert, and a psychiatric one at that. I did eventually venture to speak to defend the concept of expertise and that having expertise is not necessarily the same as relating as an authoritarian expert.

Unfortunately, like power and authority, experts and expertise conjure up images of control and coercion. This is unfortunate because it leads to generalisations and unthinking condemnation, when in fact what we should be doing is defining more closely our terms and developing broader views of these concepts. For those aspiring to promote the person-centred approach within health care settings this is vital. According to Mearns and Thorne, person-centred practitioners are often ambivalent towards the exercise of power, and in our 'desire not to *abuse* our power, we have somehow lost the ability to *exercise* our power' (2000, p. 217, original italics). I think person-centred practitioners have possibly alienated themselves and widened the gap between themselves and other mental health professionals by their over-zealous attack on experts and excessive cautiousness in using their own power and expertise.

As a psychiatrist, I do think of myself as someone who has expertise, which by definition means that I am an expert in my field. I have acquired knowledge and understanding in the fields of medicine and psychiatry throughout my training, making me an expert certainly in terms of being an information resource. As I gain experience I become more adept at applying judgements to different situations and knowing how to apply my knowledge. I believe it takes expertise to grasp situations intuitively, and to be able to handle large quantities of data and know what is most important to know. Developing expertise (which is not equivalent to amassing qualifications) leads to the increasing ability to take responsibility and to work autonomously, as well as knowing one's limits, intellectually and emotionally. Considerable expertise is required from mental health professionals to know their way around the mental health system and to know how to make it work best for patients (which is often based on informal conversations with the right people at the right time, rather than necessarily following 'correct' procedure and relying on bureaucratic referral processes). Attending to the quality of relationships with patients and colleagues, communicating effectively, developing reflective capacities and the ability to tease out ethical dilemmas and value conflicts, are all areas in which I regard myself as having some degree of expertise, as well as knowing my limitations. I could add more, but of those things I have just highlighted, many, I am sure, would be recognised by person-centred therapists as being important qualities and aspects of their work also. I do not think it is helpful, or even honest, to deny one's expertise, whether as a psychiatrist or person-centred therapist. However, what being an expert should not imply or lead to, is a sense of superiority, or encounters with other people – colleagues, patients or clients – in which there develops an oppressive imbalance of power. Being controlling and authoritarian in manner and attitude should not be the inevitable consequence of being an expert, although unfortunately it often is.

It is increasingly recognised that the patient is also an expert – an expert concerning their own experience of symptoms or illness – and therefore needs to have more say in the care they receive. This is another example of the cultural change in health care in recent years. In 1999 the government set up a national Expert Patients Programme, as part of its vision for a patient-centred NHS, which has made recommendations on managing chronic physical illnesses (DH, 2001). In mental health the government also formally consults service-users and seems to seek 'user-involvement' in developing services. However, as noted by Pilgrim (2005) professionals and managers usually determine which part of any consulta-tion they want to take on board and dictate the terms of user-involvement, thus remaining in a position of power and decision-making. Service-users can also play an important role in the teaching and training of psychiatrists (Ikkos, 2003) and other mental health professionals, especially addressing issues of power (Diamond and Hardy, 2004).

The person-centred approach would of course go a lot further, saying that not only is the patient the expert about his or her own experience (his or her feelings, thoughts, fears and hopes), but that he or she is likely to know best concerning what he or she needs in terms of help. Certainly this is a key assumption made in the situation of person-centred counselling and psychotherapy. However, it is important to stay mindful of the fact that mental health care encompasses more than formal therapy. It is therefore an important question as to what degree patients in mental health settings should, and can, influence their own treat-ment. This will depend upon the individual, the situation and particularly upon one's point of view as a mental health professional as to a patient's right and capacity for self-determination. The fair distribution of NHS resources is also an important consideration in a publicly funded service. Unfortunately there are plenty of patients who do not give a second thought to these issues, whilst part of the role of a doctor, nurse or other helper is to act as gatekeeper to, and rationer of, resources that are limited and to try to establish fairness of distribution.

Person-centred theory relating to power and expertise

Another way of understanding power is the notion of *'power within'*. In this concept power is regarded as something like an energy force or a potential, in which the outcome may be creative as well as destructive. Rogers referred to the concept of 'power within' as *'personal power'* and it was a topic to which he devoted a book (1978). For Natiello, an individual with personal power has 'the ability to act effectively under one's own volition rather than under external control. It is a state wherein the individual is aware of and can act upon his or her feelings, needs, and values rather than looking to others for direction' (1987, p. 210). According to Embleton-Tudor *et al*, 'People with power have no need to control, overpower or get their own way at the expense or cost of another' (2004, p. 126).

As I see it, the person-centred attitude to power and expertise is based on two fundamental and inter-related principles of the person-centred approach. These are first, a profound belief and trust in the actualising tendency, and secondly, a commitment to the non-directive attitude. Both of these concepts are relevant to my discussion of the medical model, assessment and diagnosis (Chapter 5) and treatment (Chapter 6).

If the tendency to actualise is, according to Rogers, the innate tendency of a person to grow, heal and become all that he or she is capable of becoming, then it has to be acknowledged that this is a power or energy of extraordinary magnitude. Natiello refers to this power as an 'energy that enables persons to act, to cause or impede change, to increase their satisfaction or reach their goals' (1990, p. 269). Personally, I find it awesome to contemplate such a power and potential. However, the powerful tendency of persons to actualise requires the right environment to facilitate its expression and release. For helpers, this means providing the therapeutic conditions for constructive personality change (*see* Chapters 7 and 8). As helpers then, we do not actually give or lend power to others, we enable the other to claim, use and express what is already theirs.

It is the belief in the tendency to actualise that for many person-centred practitioners, and certainly for Rogers, leads to therapeutic practice that is non-directive. This non-directive attitude is a distinctive and distinguishing feature of traditional person-centred therapy, but to what extent it is generally appropriate in mental health settings is an important topic for discussion and debate.

Conclusion

Society seems deeply ambivalent about experts. On the one hand experts are sought after, approved of and generally rewarded with status and positions of influence and power. On the other, they can be regarded with suspicion and fear, as well as, of course, envy. I also think that we want to believe what the expert says is true, even when we doubt what they say. 'Experts who "know" are wonderfully seductive' (Heath, 2001, p. 65), and there seems to be an instinct in many of us to trust the expert.

Mental health professionals are often regarded with similar ambivalent feelings. Many patients, in my experience, want to be told by an expert what is wrong with them. We want someone to speak authoritatively about psychological issues. There is no shortage of media experts invited to make dogmatic pronouncements about the human condition, or psychological commentators on television reality shows. As has been so aptly put, 'Psychiatry runs on the same elixir that fuels the rest of medicine: a fervent wish that somebody else knows better' (Lewis, Amini and Lannon, 2000, p. 174). Yet these same experts can be deeply disliked for their knowledge and power, especially if the answers they give are not ones we agree with. The disdain for mental health experts intensifies when their opinions face us with courses of action we do not like or choices we do not want to make, particularly when facing us with having to take responsibility.

Patients receiving input from mental health services fall somewhere along a spectrum where at one end are people who hand over all power and authority to mental health professionals, and want the expert's opinion and 'answer' or 'cure'. At the other end are people who vigorously dismiss anything mental health professionals have to say about the nature of their difficulties and what could be of help (although there may be more behind such a dismissal than an anti-expert attitude). The ideal would naturally be a meeting of each other in the middle, where there could be a genuine *'power sharing'* and mutual respect for each other's expertise. This will depend upon patients being able to own their power and expertise, as well as mental health professionals being able to recognise and facilitate their expression. Too often, people with experiences of mental distress and mental illness are 'written off' and the power of recovery given little acknowledgement. As Campbell (2005, p. 77) says, 'The creation and maintenance of action groups clearly demonstrates that the capacities of people with a mental illness diagnosis have been routinely underestimated'.

I find it an immense challenge to maintain my own power and expertise, not disown it, nor inflate it to mask my own insecurities, but to use it wisely, and *at the same time* to create the climate where other people can claim their power. As the philosopher A.C. Grayling says, 'to use power gently, and for the good of others, is one of the most heroic of virtues; which is why examples of it are so rare' (2003, p. 105).

How mental health professionals view expertise and power has profound implications for psychiatric practice, such as the attitudes we bring, and how we relate, to patients, colleagues and to ourselves. It will influence our style of communicating and the type of help we offer. Concerning the bigger picture, at a political level, concepts of power, and how it is used, influence health policy and the shape of mental health services, as well as mental health legislation. These are huge issues. In my view, an awareness of power and expertise should be introduced in every mental health professional's training. Or as has been expressed even more forcefully and urgently, 'The way power is manifest in our relationships, through our institutions, interwoven with our professional status is an ethical concern that demands particular and immediate scrutiny' (Barker and Davidson, 1998, p. 16). I hope that acknowledging power imbalances as part of practising ethically, and as one of the 'Essential Shared Capabilities of the Mental Health Workforce' (DH, 2004), becomes an issue that receives genuine attention rather than one to which lip service is paid.

References

Appleby L (1992) Suicide in psychiatric patients: Risk and prevention. *British Journal of Psychiatry*, **161**: 749–758.

Barker P and Davidson B (1998) In P Barker and B Davidson (eds) *Psychiatric Nursing. Ethical Strife*. Arnold, London.

Campbell P (2005) From Little Acorns – The mental health service user movement. In A Bell and P Lindley (eds) *Beyond the Water Towers. The unfinished revolution in mental health services 1985–2005*. The Sainsbury Centre for Mental Health, London, pp. 73–82.

Department of Health (2001) *Shifting the Balance of Power within the NHS – Securing Delivery*. Department of Health, London.

Department of Health (2001) *The expert patient: a new approach to chronic disease management for the 21st century*. Department of Health, London.

Department of Health (2004) *The Ten Essential Shared Capabilities. A Framework for the Whole of the Mental Health Workforce*. Department of Health, London.

Diamond B and Hardy M (2004) Challenging the medical model. *Openmind*, **129** (September/October): 18–19.

Dineen T (1999) *Manufacturing Victims. What the psychology industry is doing to people*. Constable, London.

Embleton-Tudor L, Keemar K, Tudor K, Valentine J and Worrall M (2004) *The Person-Centred Approach. A Contemporary Introduction*. Palgrave Macmillan, Basingstoke.

Foucault M (1977) *Madness and Civilisation*. Tavistock, London.

Grayling AC (2003) *The Reason of Things. Living with Philosophy*. Phoenix, London.

Harrison T and Gray A (2003) Leadership, complexity and the mental health professional. A report on some approaches to leadership training. *Journal of Mental Health*, **12(2)**: 153–159.

Heath I (2001) A fragment of the explanation: the use and abuse of words. *Journal of Medical Ethics: Medical Humanities*, **27**: 64–69.

Heath I (2003) A Wolf in sheep's clothing: a critical look at the ethics of drug taking. *British Medical Journal*, **327**: 856–858.

Hirschhorn L (1997) *Reworking Authority. Leading and Following in the Post-Modern Organization*. MIT Press, Cambridge, MA.

Hotopf M, Wall S, Buchanan A, Wesseley S and Churchill R (2000) Changing patterns in the use of the Mental Health Act 1983 in England, 1984 to 1996. *British Journal of Psychiatry*, **176**: 479–484.

Ikkos G (2003) Engaging patients as teachers of clinical interview skills. *Psychiatric Bulletin*, **27**: 312–315.

Illich I (1995) *Limits to Medicine. Medical Nemesis: The Expropriation of Health*. Marion Boyars, London.

Johnstone L (2000) *Users and Abusers of Psychiatry. A Critical Look at Traditional Psychiatric Practice*. 2nd Edition. Brunner-Routledge, London.

Lewis T, Amini F and Lannon R (2000) *A General Theory of Love*. Vintage Books, New York.

Lynch T (2004) *Beyond Prozac. Healing mental distress*. PCCS Books, Ross-on-Wye.

Mearns D and Thorne B (2000) *Person-Centred Therapy Today. New Frontiers in Theory and Practice*. Sage, London.

Natiello P (1987) The person-centred approach: From theory to practice. *Person-centred Review*, **2(2)**: 203–216.

Natiello P (1990) The person-centred approach. Collaborative power, and cultural transformation. *Person-Centred Review*, **5(3)**: 268–286.

Natiello P (2001) *The Person-Centred Approach: A passionate presence*. PCCS Books, Ross-on-Wye.

Oxford University Press (1996) *The Oxford English Reference Dictionary*. 2nd edition. Oxford University Press, Oxford.

Persaud R (2004) Machiavelli's mask can help you gain work place power. *Hospital Doctor*, 22nd January, p. 36.

Pilgrim D (2005) Protest and Co-option. The voice of mental health service users. In A Bell and P Lindley (eds) *Beyond the Water Towers. The unfinished revolution in mental health services 1985–2005*. The Sainsbury Centre for Mental Health, London, pp. 17–26.

Proctor G (2002) *The Dynamics of Power in Counselling and Psychotherapy. Ethics, Politics and Practice*. PCCS Books, Ross-on-Wye.

Quine L (2002) Workplace bullying in junior doctors: questionnaire survey. *British Medical Journal*, **320**: 832–836.

Rogers C (1978) *Carl Rogers on Personal Power*. Constable, London.

Szmukler G (2000) Homicide inquiries. What sense do they make? *Psychiatric Bulletin*, **24**: 6–10.

Szmukler G and Holloway F (2000a) *Mental Health Law: Discrimination or Protection?* Maudsley Discussion Paper No 10. Institute of Psychiatry, London.

Szmukler G and Holloway F (2000b) Reform of the Mental Health Act. Health or Safety? *British Journal of Psychiatry*, **177**: 196–200.

Taylor PJ and Gunn J (1999) Homicide by people with mental illness: Myth and reality. *British Journal of Psychiatry*, **174**: 9–14.

Thorne B (2003) *Carl Rogers*. Sage, London.

Thornicroft G and Szmukler G (2005) The Draft Mental Health Bill in England: without principles. *Psychiatric Bulletin*, **29**: 244–247.

Chapter 4

Thinking about mental disorder: concepts and causes

'Conceptualising our mental life as some sort of enclosed world residing inside the skull does not do justice to the lived reality of human experience.'
(Bracken P and Thomas P, 2002, p. 1434)

Introduction

In this chapter I look at psychopathology and explore what traditional psychiatry and what the person-centred approach have to say about this subject. Understanding concepts and causes of mental disorder and psychopathology is necessary in order to understand what informs the processes of assessment, diagnosis and treatment. These processes are the subjects of subsequent chapters.

I begin by entering the terrains of philosophy, science and the philosophy of science. This will include the 'mind/brain problem'. These subjects tend not to receive much in-depth attention from mental health professionals, perhaps because philosophy has the ability to challenge the safe place of certainty. However, I believe it is crucial to have a basic awareness of philosophical ideas and concepts, many of which lie at the heart of many debates within psychiatry. It is my observation that much debate takes place, often heatedly, without there being a clear idea of what it is that is being debated. In other words, I think so often opportunities for constructive discussion and dialogue are wasted because of muddy thinking, sweeping generalisations and unexamined assumptions, sometimes, of course, running alongside more hidden personal and emotional agendas. Examining the concepts of disorder, illness and theories of cause also brings into focus fundamental differences between psychiatry and the person-centred approach.

The second half of this chapter examines briefly various theories of the cause of mental disorder, followed by looking at the person-centred approach to psychopathology.

The concept of mental disorder

Differences in understanding the concept of mental disorder exist not just between psychiatric professionals and those following a person-centred approach. Mental health professionals themselves represent a variety of viewpoints. Furthermore, whilst it is true that in the UK many (probably most) psychiatrists subscribe to a predominantly biomedical (scientific) view, I think it is unhelpful to make generalisations about how psychiatrists think about mental disorder. Again, whilst most psychiatrists and mental health professionals do use the term 'mental illness', there are some who both question its use and validity, and also consider the harmful social and psychological implications of such diagnoses. The Critical Psychiatry Network (not to be confused with 'anti-psychiatry') is particularly concerned with these issues (further details of this network are given at the end of this chapter).

It is ironic though, that whilst the concept of *mental disorder* lies at the heart of theory and practice in the mental health arena, there is actually no universal agreement on its definition. Wakefield, whose description is the one I am most sympathetic to, acknowledges that 'even the clearest concepts possess areas of ambiguity, indeterminacy, and vagueness, so even a correct analysis of the concept of mental disorder is unlikely to resolve all controversies' (1992, p. 385).

Wakefield arrives at an analysis of mental disorder where 'disorder lies on the boundary between the given natural world and the constructed social world' (p. 373). In other words, it has both social and biological aspects. In developing his analysis in the paper from which I quote, he also analyses and critiques other views, including that of Thomas Szasz in 'The Myth of Mental Illness' (1960).

Wakefield's definition is as follows: 'a disorder exists when the failure of a person's internal mechanisms to perform their functions as designed by nature impinges harmfully on the person's well-being as defined by social values and meanings' (p. 373).

What I value about this definition (where mechanisms can also refer to mental mechanisms) is that it brings together two major perspectives of disorder that are usually held separately – the biological and the social. It therefore seems to offer a bridge between exponents whose polarised viewpoints are often a source of antagonism. This definition acknowledges that a condition or biological entity exists (which can be regarded objectively as a dysfunction), as well as noting that a person's *well-being* is disrupted, and that his or her well-being (subjective perception of harm) is influenced by social values and meanings. It acknowledges that the point at which normal becomes abnormal depends on social norms and is, therefore, subjective. However, this approach would not appeal to those doctors and scientists who prefer to determine the existence of a condition or disorder by certain objective criteria, as is the case with standard diagnostic classificatory systems. In other words, amongst mental health professionals who undertake assessments, there is often greater emphasis placed on the first part of the definition.

Carl Rogers may well have approved of a good deal in Wakefield's definition, particularly his taking into account of both what is objective as well as subjective. Rogers, too, acknowledges both realities (although objective aspects more so in his earlier years as a psychologist), as well as the inevitable tensions between the two.

It is worth pointing out whilst considering the term mental disorder, that there is also a legal definition under the Mental Health Act 1983 of England and Wales. This is a broad definition which is not descriptive but essentially categorises four types of disorder, one of which is mental illness, a discussion of which now follows.

Illness, disease and sickness

I think it is useful to try to understand the various ways in which the terms disease, illness and sickness can be understood. *Disease* is usually regarded (at least by doctors) as a disorder of structure or function; a pathological process or deviation from a biological norm. This still often means deciding where along a continuum to place the boundary between normal and abnormal, e.g. at what point is raised blood pressure considered pathological or a disease process?

The terms illness and sickness are often used more loosely and in English dictionaries tend to be synonymous with disease. Nevertheless, these terms have been distinguished from each other. *Illness* has been defined as a subjective sense of suffering, a personal expression of distress. *Sickness* on the other hand has been referred to as a social role, with society determining who is sick and what the parameters of sickness are. A good exploration of all three terms (as well as health, healing and wholeness) is provided by Boyd (2000).

In physical medicine, using these terms to distinguish a biological process from a subjective experience and from a socially constructed condition is relatively straightforward. In the field of mental health, however, *mental illness* is the term often used to encompass all meanings and situations. Furthermore, when mental health professionals, especially psychiatrists, use the term mental illness, they are often implying a concrete abnormality or disease process, i.e. something objective rather than subjective. It was this that led Szasz to denounce the term mental illness as a myth because, according to him, no physical lesion has been, or is likely ever to be, demonstrated. According to Szasz the term 'mental illness' is really just a metaphor for an experience of disturbance and 'problems of living'. This does not deny that a person is mentally disturbed or has problems; it simply denies a physical cause. Szasz's attack on the concept of mental illness in his key paper 'The Myth of Mental Illness' (1960) was also an attack on the misuse of power by the psychiatric establishment and on how psychiatry had become an agent of social control.

Within medical circles mental illness is sometimes referred to as a 'functional' disorder because the diagnosis is based on a disorder of function, e.g. of speech or thought processes. In this way it is distinguished from an 'organic' disorder, where there is demonstrable physical pathology. Use of the term 'functional' is usually made in general hospitals as a way of saying it's 'mental not physical' or 'we haven't found a physical cause so over to the psychiatrists'.

To add to the potential confusion of this array of terms, whilst mental disorder and mental illness are often used synonymously, within mental health settings mental illness is referred to as one particular type of mental disorder, mental disorder being a broader umbrella term. Other forms of mental disorder include personality disorder, mental disorder secondary to known physical pathology such as a brain injury (organic disorder with psychological consequences), and developmental disorder such as autism, Asperger's syndrome and disorders that come under the heading 'mental impairment'. Interestingly, in the Mental Health Act 1983, mental illness is not defined, under the belief that this is a matter of clinical judgement in the individual case.

What usually distinguishes mental illness from other forms of mental disorder is that it has a point of onset, even if this is often hard to identify precisely. Thus, a person was functioning well before experiencing the illness and can recover to how they were previously, although in reality many mental illnesses develop into chronic conditions that will inevitably impact upon personality and longer-term functioning.

Personality disorder, however, describes a condition in which a personality has developed in a disordered way during the period when personality development is at its most active. According to DSM IV (2000) it is 'an enduring pattern of inner experience and behavior that deviates markedly from the expectations of the individual's culture, is pervasive and inflexible, has an onset in adolescence or early adulthood, is stable over time, and leads to distress or impairment' (p. 685).

Inner experience refers to thinking and feeling, both of which directly influence behaviour. Most definitions regard personality or personality traits as representing characteristics of a person that, because they are enduring and relatively inflexible, lead to consistent patterns of behaviour throughout a person's lifetime. Personality disorder would then translate as consistent patterns of *disordered* behaviour throughout that person's life.

Personality disorder is a controversial diagnosis. There are many reasons for this. It requires grappling with the abstract concept of personality, and how to conceptualise personality traits. DSM IV (2000) defines personality traits as 'enduring patterns of perceiving, relating to, and thinking about the environment and oneself that are exhibited in a wide range of social and personal contexts' (p. 686).

There are also disagreements about how much personality is able to change. Rogers' view (and mine) is a more optimistic one. He sees personality as being in a continuous process of development, rather than as a fixed entity (described in Chapter 2). This means that there is potential for a person to undergo profound personality change and development, even in later years. Another problematic issue is that a subjective judgement is required as to what a 'normal' personality is in order to assess whether the resulting behaviour is normal or abnormal. It is usually society that decides what is normal and acceptable behaviour. Naturally, society influences mental health professionals who also make subjective judgements as to what constitutes 'clinically significant distress or impairment' (American Psychiatric Association, 2000, p. 686).

In mental health settings attempts are regularly made to distinguish between mental illness and personality disorder. One of the main reasons for this is the view that mental illness is often generally considered more straightforward and worthwhile attempting to treat than personality disorder. Given that the 'treatability' of personality disorder is debated within psychiatry in the first place (Moran, 1999), attempting to provide treatment (whatever treatment means) is often thought of as not a worthwhile use of scarce resources. One of my frequent irritations is hearing colleagues refer to only mental illness as a genuine disorder, and therefore more worthy of attention, excluding personality disorder from equal consideration. This is regardless of the political issue of which service, or none, should be charged with providing such attention, and I acknowledge that mental health services are currently poorly equipped to respond helpfully and therapeutically to people with damaged personalities. These attitudes (often prejudices and moral judgements) are reflected sometimes by questions such as 'Does this person have an illness or is it just personality?' It is the 'just' that is so telling.

For many person-centred practitioners, definitions and classifications of mental disorder might seem irrelevant, for reasons that will be explored later. However, for person-centred practitioners working in health settings in particular, it is worth being aware and having some understanding of these issues because they lie at the heart of all sorts of value judgements about people with mental disorder. Understanding the distinctions that are made, for example, between mental illness and personality disorder, helps to understand some of the influences on allocation of resources and structuring of services.

Material realities and the triumph of scientific objectivity

Having initially undergone a general medical training, psychiatrists are schooled in scientific thinking and methods, in the importance of objectivity, of logic, and of distinguishing between theories and observable facts. They are trained in what is known by philosophers as *logical positivism*. This is the paradigm that, despite the existence of other paradigms within psychiatry, currently predominates within NHS mental health services. It is a paradigm based on objective observation and operational criteria. It is mechanistic and it influences, for example, both neuroscience and cognitive and behavioural psychology. In considering paradigms a definition may be useful here. One such, regarding science, defines the concept of a paradigm as 'a constellation of shared assumptions, beliefs and values that unite a scientific community' (Okasha, 2002, p. 81). In short, a paradigm refers to a particular outlook.

In the last fifteen years or so there has been a growing interest in philosophy within the psychiatric profession (Fulford, Morris *et al*, 2003), despite the 1990s famously being declared 'The Decade of the Brain' (Library of Congress, 1990). However, within the medical profession (which includes psychiatrists), philosophy, like ethics, has some way to go in shaking off the way it is often rather disparagingly referred to as a 'soft science', attitudes that can become embedded at medical school. This antipathy towards philosophy partly reflects, I think, a deep attachment to scientific certainties. As Tana Dineen so aptly puts it, 'society is easily convinced of the value of anything characterised as science' (1999, p. 87), and the same could be said of many mental health professionals, particularly psychiatrists. Within psychiatry, it would of course be more accurate to refer to the 'myth' of scientific certainty, as applied to such theories as illness being caused by a chemical imbalance. References to chemical imbalances should be in terms of a working hypothesis, albeit a good one.

If this sounds as though I am rejecting science let me be clear that I am not. It is very unfortunate that people given to questioning the claims of science are accused of being 'anti-science'. What I question is what could be called 'scientific imperialism' – the idea that science can answer all the important questions about human beings. I object to the way 'society treats scientists as experts, whose opinions are regularly sought on matters of importance and for the most part accepted without question' (Okasha, 2002, p. 121). And nowhere is it truer than in Medicine that 'if someone accuses you of behaving "unscientifically", they are almost certainly criticising you' (Okasha, 2002, p. 121).

What I wish to highlight is the fact that psychiatrists are initiated into the scientific community where philosophical approaches and alternative languages are not particularly well received. Little encouragement is given to questioning scientific values and many psychiatrists learn to pronounce such scientific 'truths' in dogmatic fashion.

A good example of such dogmatic pronouncements concerning mental events is as follows:

'"You", your joys and your sorrows, your memories and your ambitions, your sense of personal identity and free will, are in fact no more than the behaviour of a vast assembly of nerve cells and associated molecules' (Crick, 1994, p. 3).

Francis Crick, although not a psychiatrist but an eminent biologist and Nobel Prize winner for his work on decoding the DNA molecule, nevertheless illustrates a type of thinking prevalent within psychiatry. This is the assumption that all mental life can be explained and understood *solely* in terms of biological processes, and further, that these processes can be understood by taking them apart to examine them.

Two key features of science are represented in Crick's assertion. First, reality is purely physical and therefore human existence consists only of physical material, which at its minutest level consists of sub-atomic particles. This is known as *materialism*. Second, understanding physical matter and its processes is best undertaken by taking them apart and reducing them down to the simplest level in order to study them. This is *reductionism* and is the method that has led to most of the discoveries and developments within the natural sciences, as well as behavioural psychology.

Carl Rogers on science and scientific knowledge

For me it is important to recognise that Rogers does not reject logical positivism or empirical science. Having lived on a farm in his childhood he became deeply interested academically in agricultural science. He regards himself as a scientist who loves to observe, record, theorise and experiment, as the following statements testify: 'I love the precision and the elegance of science' (1968a, p. 57) and 'I value the concepts which underlie the behavioural sciences. The concern with observable behaviour, the casting of all variables in operational terms, the adequate testing of hypothesis, and the use of increasingly sophisticated design and statistics all have meaning to me' (1968a, p. 58). He acknowledges his need for order, which scientific method satisfies and which he therefore respects (1959). Many of his theories in his earlier years are the fruit of scientific methods and positivist research. In the same passage, however, Rogers also states his deep valuing of persons. As a therapist he identifies himself as 'a person who has lived deeply in human relationships'. This means, therefore, that he has a foot in both the 'world of the precise, hard scientist; and the world of the sensitive, subjective person' (1968a, p. 60), although according to O'Hara (1995), over the years he increasingly embraces his own subjective experience and shifts away from the objective approach of logical positivism.

It is perhaps his dwelling in the latter subjective world of feelings, values and intuition that led Rogers to question the nature of science and how scientific 'truths' are arrived at, as the following passage demonstrates:

> '... it appears to me that though there may be such a thing as objective truth, I can never know it; all I can know is that some statements appear to me subjectively to have the qualifications of objective truth. Thus there is no such thing as Scientific Knowledge; there are only individual perceptions of what appears to each person to be such knowledge' (1959, p. 192).

Thorne points out that 'this commitment to scientific enquiry allied to a basic ambivalence about its ultimate efficacy constitutes a somewhat uneasy tension which persisted at some level throughout Rogers' life and continues to be observable among person-centred therapists since his death' (2003, p. 11). I share that ambivalence and tension, as well as Rogers' increasing desire to explore ways of transcending science and going beyond it, which may well lead into territories one might call spiritual and mystical.

Rogers is also concerned with what he sees as the depersonalisation and dehumanisation of the individual, to which he believes behavioural science contributes. He dislikes how science treats people as objects and he objects to science, as he sees it, leading 'in the direction of reductionism – to more and more minute elements which deny the overall experience which frequently is the very significant one' (1968b, p. 162). He is concerned with the philosophical puzzle – paradox even – for behavioural science to be objective without treating people as objects (O'Hara, 1995).

In short, Rogers views science as leaving out the person and the personal, of doing things *to* people rather than *for* them. He wants the behavioural sciences to see the 'subjective human being; not simply as a machine; not simply as an object or a determined sequence of cause and effect' (1968a, p. 71). He sees science as limited in its apprehending of subjective reality and in contributing to the larger field of knowledge, particularly science relating to the understanding of human beings. He wants to preserve the values of logical positivism and for science to find a way of apprehending the subjective (1959).

I very much relate to the conflicts with which Rogers wrestles in his appreciation of objective positivist science *and* the subjective world of feelings and values. I also relate to his strong objection to dogmatism, something which empirical science has a strong tendency towards. Finally, I share the observation and belief that 'a curious correlation has prevailed between scientific rigor and coldness: the more factually grounded a model of the mind, the more alienating' (Lewis, Amini and Lannon, 2000, p. 10). This statement by three psychiatrists in the USA is a contemporary observation of science and its attempt to understand mental phenomena. The problem with neuroscience, the current preoccupation of psychiatry, as I see it, is that it can depersonalise human beings in ways similar to the behavioural sciences of Rogers' day.

Mind, brain and the 'mind/brain problem'

Thinking about the concept of mind has a significant place in the history and development of psychiatry. Furthermore, how the mind is understood, given our current knowledge of the brain, is a subject that continues to engage philosophers, psychologists and scientists. However, given that this is such a fundamental 'problem', it is staggering how relatively little it is considered in everyday mental health practice and in the thinking of and debates between mental health professionals. This is regrettable. Our questions about the mind, such as whether it is a physical substance, an aspect of the brain, or a concept outside the realm of science, whether the brain and mind are separate or inter-related, constitute, in my opinion, the foundations of what mental health professionals do. How we view the mind and the brain acts as a guide to the way we respond to people in various forms of mental distress, including the language we use – scientific, psychological or spiritual.

One of the most influential Western thinkers on the subject of mind was the French philosopher René Descartes (1596–1650), who lived at a time when science as we now know it was born, heralding the era of modernism. He proposes that human beings consist of a physical (material) body and a non-physical mind. Mental states – activities such as thinking and feeling – according to Descartes, occur in the non-material mind (also referred to as the soul) and it is these that determine the identity of the 'person'. Although he regards the mind and body as connected (initially via the pineal gland in the brain, although he later abandons this idea), he also believes that the mind could operate independently from the body, including after death. In other words, the 'I' could exist without the body.

So-called 'Cartesian dualism' – one of the legacies of Descartes – refers to the belief that there are two separate, although connected, entities (or 'substances') known as body and mind. This conceptual 'splitting' continues to exist in the way human beings both conceptualise and are conceptualised. We tend often to think in terms of 'either/or' rather than 'both/and'. How often do people say, or imply, that there is nothing wrong physically because 'it's all in the mind'? Is it mental illness or personality disorder? Or, according to Szasz, is it brain disease or problems of living? Even the medical specialties support this false demarcation, with neurologists dealing with the brain and psychiatrists the mind.

However, the progress of science, taking over as it has from religion since the 1600s in explaining the natural world, has also had a pivotal role in the mind/body debate. In fact, in many scientific circles (particularly the natural sciences) the mind is actually now regarded as somewhat of a myth, or purely an abstract concept, and not the 'substance' Descartes regards it to be. Mental activities are viewed as the result of physical processes in the brain (materialism again – the belief that in time we will be able to explain the complexities of mental life by the laws of chemistry and physics). The concept of mind can still be used, but materialists would refer to mind processes as essentially brain processes under another name. Incidentally, in the East and in complementary medical approaches there is far less mind/body dualism and greater holistic integration, although this does not imply that the mind and the brain are one and the same.

As said earlier, this 'brain/mind' debate has profound consequences for the practice of psychiatry, underpinning as it does our understanding of human beings, concepts of person-hood, consciousness, the nature of mental experiences including how they become disturbed (psychopathology), and views about morality, choice, autonomy, free will and responsibility. All this, in turn, influences the processes of assessment, diagnosis and treatment. Given how fundamental these ideas are, it is amazing to me that there is so little formal education and discussion on this subject for mental health professionals, including psychiatrists. My own knowledge and understanding of these philosophical ideas, which are admittedly only very basic, stem from my own reading and researching that has grown out of my own interest.

Causes of mental disorder

I turn now to the topic of what causes mental disorder, although rather than use the word 'cause', it would be more helpful and accurate to think in terms of what *influences the development of* mental disorder. As there are many explanatory models (a model being a conceptual framework), this can therefore only be a brief summary. However, perhaps the key point to emphasise at the outset is the fact that there are currently many theories and models of what influences the development of mental disorder. This partly reflects our current lack of knowledge and uncertainty about what constitutes mental processes, and simply how much of our understanding of human beings and their behaviours remains a mystery.

Within psychiatry there are several camps into which many psychiatrists firmly place themselves, whilst other psychiatrists may loosely affiliate themselves with all the various camps. Psychiatrists who identify themselves as neuroscientists would explain mental processes in biological terms, and are likely to see the brain and the mind as essentially the same. Other psychiatrists might be more interested in psychological models, of which there are many. Others still are more interested in social perspectives. Within psychiatry then, there is not one all-encompassing explanatory theory of human mental experience, behaviour and mental disorder. This can result in a kind of conceptual 'pick 'n' mix' leading to controversies and conflicts concerning which conceptual models to embrace, both amongst psychiatrists and between psychiatrists and other mental health professionals. Tensions arise particularly when deciding which management or treatment approach to adopt, which depends upon how mental disorder is first conceptualised.

The disease model

The *disease model* understands mental disorder to be a physical disorder of structure or function. In this model, mental events are seen as brain events. Biological (physical) factors considered include brain anatomy, physiology and biochemistry, genetic influences on these and also the effects of drugs on brain processes. In the absence of observable or detectable physical pathology such as a brain tumour or infection, the most keenly pursued theories of mental disorder concern brain biochemistry and theories of chemical imbalance of neurotransmitters, these being the chemical messengers between brain cells. Of course, the pharmaceutical industry reinforces the disease model since it is their products that aim to 'correct' chemical imbalance.

Although the influence of the pharmaceutical industry, particularly on doctors, can make it easy to be cynical about the disease model, it would be short-sighted to reject biological explanations. Mental processes such as our emotions and thinking do involve nerve cells and their connections. The brain is not for nothing a vast complex of a hundred billion cells through which electric currents travel and which communicate with each other chemically. Neuroscience is increasingly gaining insights into aspects of cognition and emotions. Imaging techniques are also showing us how our experience both shapes and is being shaped by developing brain structures. In other words, experience moulds the brain and its connections. Even though the young brain is the most 'plastic', neural connections are subject to on-going development throughout a person's life (Eisenberg, 2000; Lewis, Amini and Lannon, 2000). Needless to say, this has implications for how we view personality development and change.

Where does our genetic heritage fit into all this? If genes establish the template, experience and the environment then interact with the template to determine which genes are switched on and off. Or, as Amini, Lewis and Lannon put it, 'the genetic lottery may determine the cards in your deck, but experience deals the hand you can play' (2000, pp. 152–153).

Already I have moved into the other major influence on mental processes and disorder. This is the realm of psychological factors, a major part of our 'experience' of life.

Psychological models

We talk about 'the psychological' so easily, but what does this ubiquitous term mean when thinking about the development of disorder? Like so many terms, it is really an umbrella term, and so much so that it is almost meaningless, other than meaning 'not physical' and something other than a straightforward brain-based theory. Essentially, 'psychological' relates to the mind or mental realm, whatever we might mean by the term mind.

There are then, many psychological explanatory models. Within psychiatry the most prominent are *cognitive* theories with their focus upon beliefs and thinking patterns as the determinants of disordered mental states and behaviour. Related *behavioural* models draw on, for example, the conditioning theories of Pavlov and Skinner. *Psychodynamic (psychoanalytical)* theories have developed from the time of Sigmund Freud and, to a lesser extent within psychiatry, Carl Jung. There are many psychoanalytical schools of thought and the object relations theorists such as Melanie Klein and Donald Winnicot have also been influential. *Humanistic* psychological models and theories such as transactional analysis and the person-centred approach receive much less attention in the training of mental health professionals, as do *existential* perspectives. *Family systems theory* has some influence, influenced as it is by social perspectives.

Social models

Social dimensions of mental disorder consider such influences as the development of dysfunctional interpersonal relationships (within families, communities and societies), employment, the roles individuals play within society, poverty and other environmental factors. Interest in this area shifts the location of the disorder from within the individual to their environment and its power structures, social and cultural values, expectations and norms.

The biopsychosocial model

Attempts have been made to bring together the various theories and models that have been used to understand the development of mental disorder, and in so doing, attempt to see the individual in as holistic a way as possible. Mental health professionals who attempt to take this approach may do so as a way of evading the clutches of reductionism and logical positivism.

The biopsychosocial model was proposed by George Engel (1980), a psychiatrist, although his ideas are originally expressed by Adolf Meyer, another psychiatrist, working in America in the first half of the twentieth century, whose work is now largely forgotten (Double, 2002). Meyer stresses the need for psychiatry to attend to the patient as a person, whilst not rejecting biological aspects of disturbance. A contemporary view has been expressed by Bracken and Thomas who believe that 'conceptualising our mental life as some sort of enclosed world residing inside the skull does not do justice to the lived reality of human experience' (2002, p. 1434).

Neither Engel's biopsychosocial model nor Meyer's psychobiological model are attempts to provide a meta-theory of the development of mental disorder, and because of this these models do not offer a coherent guide to treatment. (Perhaps the term 'model' here is not very useful if what we mean by model is a simplified framework to explain phenomena.) Furthermore, because these approaches do not offer a neat integration of theories, they do not easily lend themselves to research. Perhaps this is partly why in practice often lip service only is paid to the biopsychosocial model.

The reality is that it can be a struggle to conceptualise the connections or relationship between biology (our nerve cells and chemicals), our psyche or mind (assuming here that the mind isn't just another metaphor for brain and therefore really a biological entity) and our social context. Are these various factors and influences like links in a chain? How do we integrate the data we receive when assessing people in mental and emotional distress? Should we be so interested in cause and explanation in the first place, rather than focusing upon the person's subjective experience for no other reason than to convey understanding? Understanding here does not mean the intellectual understanding of cause but something different. The terms 'explaining' and 'understanding' are explored in the next chapter.

In my opinion, it seems too difficult at present for psychiatry and mental health services to work with numerous explanatory theories and from multiple paradigms. Kuhn, who popularised the term paradigm, argues that paradigmatic differences cannot be reconciled (Kuhn, 1963). The possibility of inhabiting more than one paradigm at the same time is an interesting philosophical question.

More often than not psychiatry adheres to disease theories because, as has been suggested by Eisenberg, it can 'seek professional respectability by adhering to a reductionistic model of mental disorder' (1986, p. 500). Psychiatrists, by being able to focus on physical aspects, order investigations, diagnose and work from the medical model, can stand on equal terms with their medical colleagues. Double also suggests that the psychobiological model is not tolerated because 'refocusing psychiatry on the patient as a person emphasises the uncertainty of psychiatric practice' (2002, p. 900). However, there are also powerful political reasons for pursuing this narrow approach within psychiatry, and gross shortage of resources is a significant factor. When medications are one of the few things mental health services have to offer, there will be a tendency to justify their use by focusing on chemical imbalance theories of disorder. If there were greater availability of psychological therapies, there would probably be more discussion of psychological factors in the aetiology of mental disorder. This is an example of how resources, policy and politics influence the thinking and researching towards understanding mental disorder and how politics influences paradigms.

Given the relative powerlessness mental health professionals experience in terms of influencing societal structures and values, family relationships, employment, poverty and the epidemic of children and adolescents growing up with feelings of worthlessness, shame and anxiety, it is tempting to ignore or only briefly acknowledge these social issues. It is easier to influence brain chemicals through medication than family structures and societal values.

Predispositions and triggers

Another way in which it can be helpful to conceptualise the development of mental disorder is to think in terms of predisposing factors (e.g. biological ones such as genetic inheritance or brain structure and psychological ones such as personality) and triggering (or precipitating) factors, such as life events and major stresses. Added to this are perpetuating factors which can maintain states of mental distress and are often a person's social circumstances. It is clear to see from this that the word 'cause' is a very broad term (covering both 'nature' and 'nurture') that is often used rather simplistically. As well as describing 'influences' on the development of mental disorder, 'association' might also be a term better suited to explaining the development of disorder. For example, depression can often be associated with experiences of loss.

The person-centred approach to psychopathology

The person-centred approach has been accused of having no theory of psycho-pathology. This assumption is unfair, particularly given the attention Rogers gave to the origins of psychological disturbance in his personality theory. Joseph and Worsley have recently edited a book with the title 'Person-Centred Psycho-pathology' (2005a), focusing exclusively on this subject. What is probably the case, however, is that most person-centred practitioners are generally more comfortable talking about mental *health*, growth and development potential of human beings than mental *illness* and psychopathology.

The spirit of the person-centred approach tends to question the conceptual validity of mental illness and is often critical of what it perceives as the over-emphasis on the disease model in understanding mental distress. There is a range of reasons why person-centred practitioners align themselves with opponents of illness models and prefer concepts such as 'problems of living'. Disagreements about theoretical models of cause are only one of them. Other concerns are the issues of power, stigma, medicalisation and the ethos and treatment approaches within mental health services which models of psychopathology directly influ-ence. It is, however, perfectly possible to challenge and criticise psychiatry on these issues whilst nevertheless accepting the language and concept of mental illness, as is the case for many user groups and mental health charities. It is sometimes unclear what one is arguing against given how many of these issues overlap.

Rogers is not against medication, nor does he avoid using language that classifies disorders broadly into neurosis and psychosis. (Psychosis and neurosis are broad terms to describe mental phenomena and are not in themselves diagnostic categories.) He also led a research project using the person-centred approach amongst an in-patient population of people diagnosed with schizo-phrenia – the so-called 'Wisconsin Project' (Rogers, Gendlin *et al*, 1967).

What is true is that Rogers' theory is not a specific illness or disorder theory. His theories of mental disturbance are part of his overall theory of personality when he is considering incongruence, defence processes and the process of breakdown and disorganisation (Rogers, 1959). It is also true that his theory does not help much in understanding the various manifestations of mental disturbance, i.e., why some people become psychotic and others develop neurotic responses, or why someone might be predisposed to a generalised anxiety disorder and another to obsessive-compulsive disorder. Instead, he is more interested in what experiences mean for people, more in the 'how' than in the 'why' of mental experience. He is not interested in categorising or classifying disturbance. Not only does classifying disorder tend to depersonalise people, but also his approach to therapy is actually the same regardless of diagnosis. The person-centred approach to therapy as Rogers formulates it is not disorder-specific and therefore leaves little rationale for the helper or therapist using diagnostic categories.

However, concepts of psychopathology are now receiving more attention within the person-centred community, particularly in mainland Europe, evidenced by Joseph and Worsley's book (2005a). Several practitioners have become known in the person-centred world for work on particular forms of psychopathology or problem areas. Among the most notable are Gary Prouty and his work on 'psychological contact' and the development of 'Pre-therapy' (*see* Chapter 9). This is an approach that aims to establish psychological contact with people whose ability to make or maintain psychological contact is impaired, for example, by psychosis, dissociative states or dementia (Prouty, Van Werde and Pörtner, 2002). Margaret Warner is known for her work on 'processing' – the way human beings make sense of their experiences and how experiences of disturbance are mentally processed. The different types of process she describes are fragile, dissociated and psychotic process (Warner, 2000; 2005). There have been other areas of development in, for example, post traumatic stress disorder (Joseph, 2003; 2005), and alcohol problems (Bryant-Jefferies, 2001).

Some of these developments have caused tensions within the person-centred community. Some practitioners who remain faithful to the 'classical' person-centred approach might regard those practitioners developing models of psychopathology as forming an unholy alliance with traditional psychiatry and the medical model, although I think many would be in favour of constructive dialogue. However, the counter argument is that the person-centred approach needs to be able to demonstrate its effectiveness to those purchasing mental health services. Practitioners therefore need to learn the language of psychiatry at least, in order to gain a foothold within services that are currently dominated by neuroscience and the reductionism of cognitive-behavioural and other evidence-based approaches.

I personally find this a difficult dilemma and would not want the person-centred approach to compromise its fundamental values and philosophy and allow itself to be contaminated by the current culture of mental health services, which are in desperate need of being humanised and which I believe the person-centred approach has the potential to do. Rogers, no doubt, would want the person-centred approach to psychopathology to develop organically in the way that his own theory and practice developed. It may be that forming alliances with such movements as the Critical Psychiatry Network and Positive Psychology (the latter being a new movement among psychologists (Seligman, 2003; Joseph and Worsley, 2005b)) will enable a model of psychopathology to be developed without being overly influenced by the medical model and preoccupations with diagnosis.

Conclusion

It has been salutary to realise through writing this chapter and my researching for it just how many assumptions I had previously made, and not thought to question, about the whole bedrock of theory upon which my practice as a psychiatrist is based. It has also become clear what a minefield of terminology one is required to negotiate in order to understand how mental health services work. Furthermore, underlying many of these terms are concepts that are abstract and potentially confusing. Nevertheless, mental health professionals use language in a way that often implies unquestioned acceptance of its validity and usefulness. Dogmatic assertions on the supremacy of science are, in my opinion, harmful. But to wholly condemn science and its methods would be equally misguided.

The challenge as I see it is to understand the many 'frames of reference' (in person-centred terms) and understand the many different languages used within mental health services. Rogers is a good role model in the way he attempts to communicate across paradigms. I believe it is also very important to know as much as possible about our own theoretical and philosophical leanings and how much we agree and identify with the language we use. As Coulson says, 'If each scientist doesn't philosophise explicitly he will philosophise implicitly, and badly' (1968, p. 149). This must surely apply to all of us whose work is of a helping nature, whether within an organisation and as part of our professional role or in other contexts outside of our work places.

References

American Psychiatric Association (2000) *Diagnostic and Statistical Manual of Mental Disorders.* 4th Edition. Text Revision. American Psychiatric Association, Washington, DC.

Boyd K (2000) Disease, illness, sickness, health, healing and wholeness: exploring some elusive concepts. *Journal of Medical Ethics: Medical Humanities,* **26**: 9–17.

Bracken P and Thomas P (2002) Time to move beyond the mind-body split. *British Medical Journal,* **325**: 1433–1434.

Bryant-Jefferies R (2001) *Counselling the Person Beyond the Alcohol Problem.* Jessica Kingsley Publishers, London.

Coulson W (1968) On Science and Knowledge. In W Coulson and C Rogers (eds) *Man and the Science of Man.* Charles Merrill Publishing Company, Columbus, Ohio, pp. 132–150.

Crick F (1994) *The Astonishing Hypothesis: The Scientific Search for the Soul.* Simon and Schuster, London.

Dineen T (1999) *Manufacturing Victims. What The Psychology Industry Is Doing To People.* Constable, London.

Double D (2002) The limits of psychiatry. *British Medical Journal,* **324**: 900–904.

Eisenberg L (1986) Mindlessness and Brainlessness in Psychiatry. *British Journal of Psychiatry,* **148**: 497–508.

Eisenberg L (2000) Is psychiatry more mindful or brainier than it was a decade ago? *British Journal of Psychiatry,* **176**: 1–5.

Engel G (1980) The clinical application of the biopsychosocial model. *American Journal of Psychiatry,* **137**: 535–544.

Fulford KWM, Morris K, Sadler J and Stanghellini G (2003) Past improbable, future possible: the renaissance in philosophy and psychiatry. In KWM Fulford, K Morris,

J Sadler and G Stanghellini (eds) *Nature and Narrative. An introduction to the new philosophy of psychiatry*. Oxford University Press, Oxford, pp. 1–41.

Joseph S (2003) Person-centred approach to understanding posttraumatic stress. *Person-Centred Practice*, **11**: 70–75.

Joseph S (2005) Understanding Post-Traumatic Stress from the Person-Centred Perspective. In S Joseph and R Worsley (eds) *Person-Centred Psychopathology. A Positive Psychology of Mental Health*. PCCS Books, Ross-on-Wye, pp. 190–201.

Joseph S and Worsley R (eds) (2005a) *Person-Centred Psychopathology. A Positive Psychology of Mental Health*. PCCS Books, Ross-on-Wye.

Joseph S and Worsley R (2005b) A Positive Psychology of Mental Health: The person-centred perspective. In S Joseph and R Worsley (eds) *Person-Centred Psychopathology. A Positive Psychology of Mental Health*. PCCS Books, Ross-on-Wye, pp. 348–357.

Kuhn T (1963) *The Structure of Scientific Revolutions*. University of Chicago Press, Chicago.

Lewis T, Amini F and Lannon R (2000) *A General Theory of Love*. Vintage Books, New York.

Library of Congress (1990) *Project on the Decade of the Brain*. www.loc.gov/loc/brain/

Moran P (1999) *Should Psychiatrists Treat Personality Disorders?* Maudsley Discussion Paper No 7. Institute of Psychiatry, London.

O'Hara M (1995) Carl Rogers: Scientist and Mystic. *Journal of Humanistic Psychology*, **35(4)**: 40–53.

Okasha S (2002) *Philosophy of Science. A Very Short Introduction*. Oxford University Press, Oxford.

Prouty G, Van Werde D and Pörtner M (2002) *Pre-Therapy. Reaching contact-impaired clients*. PCCS Books, Ross-on-Wye.

Rogers C (1959) A theory of therapy, personality and interpersonal reationships as developed in the client-centred framework. In S Koch (ed) *Psychology: A study of a science: Vol. 3. Formulations of the person and the social context*. McGraw-Hill, New York, pp. 184–256.

Rogers C, Gendlin E, Kiesler D and Truax C (1967) *The Therapeutic Relationship with Schizophrenics*. The University of Wisconsin Press, Wisconsin.

Rogers C (1968a) Some Thoughts Regarding the Current Presuppositions of the Behavioral Sciences. In W Coulson and C Rogers (eds) *Man and the Science of Man*. Charles Merrill Publishing Company, Columbus, Ohio, pp. 55–72.

Rogers C (1968b) On Science and Truth. In W Coulson and C Rogers (eds) *Man and the Science of Man*. Charles Merrill Publishing Company, Columbus, Ohio, pp. 152–168.

Seligman M (2003) Positive Psychology: Fundamental assumptions. *The Psychologist*, **55**: 5–14.

Szasz T (1960) The Myth of Mental Illness. *The American Psychologist*, **15**: 113–118.

Thorne B (2003) *Carl Rogers*. Sage, London.

Wakefield J (1992) The Concept of Mental Disorder. On the Boundary Between Biological Facts and Social Values. *American Psychologist*, **47(3)**: 373–388.

Warner M (2000) Person-Centred Therapy at the Difficult Edge: a Developmentally Based Model of Fragile and Dissociated Process. In D Mearns and B Thorne *Person-Centred Therapy Today. New Frontiers in Theory and Practice*. Sage, London, pp. 144–171.

Warner M (2005) A Person-Centred View of Human Nature, Wellness, and Psychopathology. In S Joseph and R Worsley (eds) *Person-Centred Psychopathology. A Positive Psychology of Mental Health*. PCCS Books, Ross-on-Wye, pp. 91–109.

Further references

Critical Psychiatry Network www.criticalpsychiatry.co.uk
Positive Psychology www.positivepsychology.org

Chapter 5

What is wrong with me? Assessment, diagnosis and the medical model

'If one looks at the nature of human nature, psychodiagnosis barely scratches the surface of a person's essence, that person's inner world of feelings, beliefs, perceptions, values, and attitudes ...'

(Boy, 2002, p. 388)

Introduction

In the previous chapter I discussed the disease model, as well as other models concerning the development of mental disorder. Now I want to describe how I view the *medical model*. I want to be clear what I mean by the medical model and why I distinguish it from the disease model. The two are often used inter-changeably, particularly by critics of psychiatry, and this is unfortunate because it can cause confusion. Challenging the medical model can involve a different set of arguments to those that challenge disease theories, even though the medical model is often based on disease theories of mental disorder. I regard the medical model predominantly to describe a *way of working*. It is a *method* or *process* that has implications for the relationship between doctor and patient, or therapist and client. Thus, the medical model refers also to a particular set of power dynamics. In essence, I understand the medical model to consist of the process of assessment, diagnosis and treatment. This chapter is concerned with assessment and diagnosis and Chapter 6, treatment.

I shall also consider the contrast between the medical model and the person-centred approach and the formidable challenge for person-centred practitioners working within health services and mental health settings especially. In addition, I shall touch on phenomenology, objectivity, subjectivity and the difference between 'explaining' and 'understanding'. These issues highlight some of the tensions, certainly for me, of trying to practise psychiatry in a traditional NHS mental health setting, whilst also being sensitive to person-centred values.

Assessment

Assessment is a key aspect of the medical model, usually undertaken with a view to making a diagnosis in order to form a treatment plan or continue treating and managing the diagnosed problem or illness. It should be noted that within mental health settings there are many other types of assessment such as the increasingly prevalent risk assessment. Mental Health Act assessments are another particular type of assessment. Others include assessment for welfare benefits or accommodation schemes. When referring to assessment then, it is important to qualify what kind of assessment one is talking about because valid criticisms of one type may not apply to another. I make this point because person-centred criticisms of assessment are often unhelpfully generalised. What follows here focuses mainly on diagnostic assessments, which are often the purpose of the initial interview between the mental health professional and patient.

Assessment is essentially a process of collecting data, interpreting it and then categorising it. The psychiatric interview assessment attempts to collect two types of data. The first is the patient's 'history'. This includes such things as basic demographic data, the story of events and details leading up to the current situation, social circumstances and all other relevant factual information, as recounted by the patient, relatives or other significant parties. The second part is the 'mental state examination', which is the process of assessing thoughts, mood, perceptions, cognitive functioning and behaviours, and identifying abnormal mental phenomena such as hallucinations or suicidal thinking. In practice, history taking and mental state examination are overlapping processes. Psychiatrists are trained to use a highly structured framework of questions in an attempt to uncover symptoms and symptom clusters, the latter being a pattern of symptoms occurring together, otherwise known as 'syndromes'. The psychiatric assessment is also not complete without considering physical pathology and performing necessary physical investigations, e.g. physical examination and blood tests.

In terms of assessing symptoms or 'psychopathology' (abnormal mental phenomena), mental health professionals are taught to distinguish between what is known as the 'form' and the 'content' of the symptom. The form refers to the general characteristics and structure of the experience, for example, delusional thinking. The content is the unique characteristic of the experience for that individual; for example, the content of delusional thinking could be the idea of being watched by invisible government agents. Whilst it is the content that has particular meaning for the person and illustrates the uniqueness of their experience, it is the form that often points the psychiatrist to the diagnosis (although the above form of delusional thinking could point to any number of diagnoses).

It is often the psychiatrist's preoccupation with the form of mental experience (the commonalities of symptoms), rather than the person's individual and unique personal experience, that leads to psychiatric assessment so often being experienced by patients as impersonal and, at worst, dehumanising. Psychiatrists are taught to assess the contents of a patient's mind as though the contents were parts of a machine, for which detached objectivity is required. Sims (2003) even suggests the assessment process is analogous to a surgical procedure. Deciding when more detail is required from a patient is compared to the skill of knowing 'where to make the incision for the psychopathological operation' and where the psychiatrist 'wishes to dissect out the *form* of the patient's illness ...' (p. 32).

The diagnostic assessment is regarded as a skill, for which interviewing techniques are taught to psychiatric trainees. We learn such techniques as when to use open and closed questions. We are encouraged to 'sit down and give non-verbal cues of interest and friendliness' when preparing for the psychiatric interview (Aquilinia and Warner, 2004, p. 20). Another common technique we are taught is to let the patient have free rein for the first five minutes (to help achieve rapport) before then taking control and structuring the rest of the interview. I personally dislike such techniques, especially when conducted in a stereotyped way. They also run counter to the person-centred approach, which later chapters will highlight.

Such psychiatric interviewing and assessments also reveal the reductionist tendencies of the medical model, where psychiatrists especially, with scientific objectivity, attempt 'to assess the contents of a patient's mind' (McHugh and Slavney, 1998, p. 8). This approach leads to the caricature of the emotionally distant psychiatrist whom many patients may come to fear, rather than the warm approachable doctor interested in persons.

Another example of psychiatry's preference for the objective, reductionist approach is increasing reliance on rating scales and symptom checklists when conducting psychiatric assessments. Research, particularly when sponsored by pharmaceutical companies, relies heavily on rating scales and approaches that attempt to measure and score symptoms.

Whilst I have mostly referred to the assessment as might be conducted by a psychiatrist, it is only fair to say that in general, assessments by nurses or social workers show more interest in patients as persons and their unique story. Whilst the doctor is more interested in form, other mental health professionals tend to be more interested in content. However, some nurses are increasingly aspiring to be as scientifically reductionist as psychiatrists, straying, in my view, from the heart of nursing.

Phenomenology: being objective about the subjective

Nowhere is the detached, objective, scientific approach more required, it seems, than in assessing mental state, or so trainee psychiatrists are taught. The message I received as a junior psychiatrist was that the mark of a good clinician is the ability to discern the phenomenology (by which was meant the phenomena) of the patient by being as objective as possible. In psychiatry the term phenomenology is used for describing the method of eliciting symptoms and assessing mental state – of 'observation and categorisation of abnormal psychological events' (Sims, 2003, p. 3).

However, phenomenology is a highly complex philosophical discipline with many different strands of thinking and even different conceptions of what phenomenology is. In psychiatry it was turned into a method of investigation of psychopathology by the German psychiatrist Karl Jaspers (1883–1969). It has therefore come to be viewed in psychiatry as a scientific approach to enable classification and diagnosis, the hallmark of which is an objective and reductionist attitude. With this limited view are lost the aspects of phenomenology that, for example, are concerned with existential issues and the study of the structure of the patient's conscious mental experience from their subjective point of view. What is also lost is the aspect of phenomenology that is concerned with the meaning attached to mental experiences.

Thankfully this is not the place to explore further the subject of phenomenology because my own understanding is limited. Nevertheless, what I hope I have highlighted is the important role of objectivity, as viewed by psychiatry at least. Yet how much does the objective approach really hold out in the realm of subjective experience and meaning? My view is that psychiatry's quest to embrace reductionism and objectivity in this way is regrettable. I strongly dislike and reject the idea of someone taking my personal, subjective experience and attempting to measure or define it in a scientific and objective manner. It is unique and highly meaningful to me and only I really know something of its essence, even if others are able, perhaps, to recognise aspects of it.

It has also been argued within the arena of subatomic physics that there is no such thing as pure objectivity because the observer influences what is observed. (Heisenberg's 'uncertainty principle' states that the process of observing particles has a discreet effect on what is being measured, i.e. its position and momentum.) To me this sounds similar to what Rogers says about scientific truth. An objective assessment of a person's mental state is only one apprehension of reality and therefore cannot be *the* reality. Furthermore, claims of objective science being value-free are misplaced. Our biases and prejudices colour our psychiatric assessments, as do all our preoccupations and feelings. Unfortunately it would seem that this is given little attention in the training of mental health professionals, judging by the way the findings of assessment are frequently presented as *the* reality, uninfluenced by our own subjective experiencing. There is little encouragement of mental health professionals to develop a thorough self-awareness and reflect on how their own mental states influence the assessment of the mental states of others. I believe this lack of commitment to self-awareness is short-sighted and does a profound disservice, and sometimes even damage, to patients.

Within the person-centred approach, phenomenology does not refer to a method of categorising mental experiences. It focuses on a person's subjective experience, as it is, without trying to impose a preconceived framework, define or explain it. The person-centred approach is concerned with how human beings experience the world and construct meaning and is influenced here by the existential branch of phenomenology and existential philosophers such as Kierkegaard, whom Rogers quotes. More particularly, the person-centred approach is interested in the subjective reality of the patient more for its own sake and as an *expression* of empathy, rather than *using* empathy to get at the subjective experience in order to diagnose, as psychiatrists are taught.

There are few other situations than when conducting the assessment interview, in which I feel more the tensions inherent in my role as a psychiatrist and my valuing of the person-centred approach. I feel acutely the dilemma of how far to pursue with objectivity the study of a patient's mental state with the goal of formulating a diagnosis, when I am naturally more drawn to giving attention to a person's experience as they present it, without seeking to delineate its characteristics or define it. How much attention do I give to the form and how much to the content of mental experience? How much am I simply the observer and categoriser of experience and how much am I engaged with the story of the other and paying attention to what is going on in the interaction and to the relationship between us?

Psychodiagnosis: the Holy Grail of psychiatry

What is this patient's diagnosis? I would be interested to know how many times in my average working day I am confronted by this question, either asked directly by colleagues or patients, or for bureaucratic purposes. A diagnosis is now required for every patient who has contact with psychiatric services, and one that comes in code form, i.e. is assigned a particular letter and number. The two most widely used classification systems are the Diagnostic and Statistical Manual of Mental Disorders, currently in its 4th edition – DSM-IV – (American Psychiatric Association, 1994) and the International Classification of Diseases, currently in its 10th edition – ICD-10 – (World Health Organization, 1992).

For patients encountering the psychiatric system then, the question of what the diagnosis is will feature prominently. It increasingly determines the treatment, management and the so-called 'care pathway'. It also determines which part of the service is responsible for that care. The design and functioning of psychiatric services are also heavily influenced by diagnosis. I have written elsewhere about the relationship between diagnosis and NHS mental health care, particularly focusing on the increasingly used category 'severe and enduring mental illness' (Freeth, 2007). The diagnosis is not just the concern of mental health professionals and the organisation, however, since many patients also clamour for a diagnosis. For many mental health charities, self-help and user groups the diagnosis also features prominently, often included in the name of the charity, such as the Manic Depression Fellowship, OCD-UK and the National Phobics Society. In other words, it is not just the preoccupation of mental health services and psychiatrists. Nevertheless, I think the pursuit of diagnosis by many mental health professionals is something similar to the search for the Holy Grail.

The issue of diagnosis is also one that creates within me numerous tensions and unease. As a psychiatrist I am certainly not alone with some of these feelings. However, along with Bracken, Thomas and Double (*see* Chapter 4) I am in a clear minority that courts hostility from colleagues for being critical of the medical model, diagnosis and the logical positivist approach, perhaps because we are seen as undermining our role and legitimacy as psychiatrists.

It is important to note that there are several categories of argument both for and against diagnosis. I have found it a complex task trying to unravel the different lines of argument that are influenced by many academic disciplines such as science, philosophy and sociology. Politics and health service design and function are now also at the forefront in shaping (some might say controlling) the debate around diagnosis. I do not intend to present a detailed analysis. Rather, I am particularly interested in what the person-centred approach has to say about diagnosis. Nevertheless, whilst there are some clear arguments opposing diagnosis based on the theory and philosophy of the person-centred approach, person-centred practitioners may also align themselves with critics of psychodiagnosis from many other camps such as the anti-psychiatry movement. Therefore, I offer a brief summary of many of the different arguments used to support the value of diagnosis, and those used to challenge and criticise it. After this I will consider more specifically person-centred perspectives.

I have identified three main categories of argument used to either support or criticise the use of psychodiagnosis. The first category is concerned with the purpose and function of diagnosis, i.e. its usefulness, reliability and validity. Second, there are arguments concerning the method of arriving at a diagnosis, i.e. the process of assessment. A third category could be the effects of diagnosis on the individual. It is also worth noting that the same argument can be used in arguing both for and against diagnosis, highlighting how much our subjective realities and philosophical position influence the way we approach these issues and what values we attach to the argument.

Arguments supporting diagnosis

These are not listed in any order of importance but are grouped into the categories I have previously identified. Although not a comprehensive list, it is clear to see that arguments in support of diagnosis are mostly concerned with the purpose and function of diagnosis and often for the convenience of mental health professionals or for political and economic expediency.

The purpose and function of diagnosis

- Classification satisfies the need for order and creates a structure for understanding.
- It enables professionals to communicate with each other, creates reference points and allows information to be summarised. It prevents the need to describe in detail and is therefore more convenient and time efficient.
- Diagnosis determines or guides treatment and management.
- It serves research purposes, much of which is involved with the development of specific drugs for specific disorders, as well as work towards being able to predict the natural course of disorders.
- In general medicine the diagnostic term often indicates the cause, although in psychiatry most diagnoses say very little, if anything, about cause.
- Diagnosis influences the use of health care resources, it enables the standardisation of treatment approaches and is the basis upon which services are organised and paid for. The current UK government's proposed 'Payment by Results' (DH, 2002) is designed around diagnosis. In other words, diagnosis has practical, political and financial purpose.

The effects of diagnosis on the individual

- For patients a diagnosis can reassure and seem to legitimise a person's mental disturbance. There is value in the naming of the type of distress.
- In recognising the commonalities of experience, patients may gain a sense of belonging and identity with other patients with the same diagnosis.

Arguments against diagnosis

Criticisms of diagnosis are more wide ranging, but many of them are concerned with the effects on the individual, both having a diagnostic label, as well as the process of assessment, particularly its depersonalising effect. Some criticisms of the method of assessment and diagnosing could also be placed in the category concerned with the effects on the individual.

The purpose and function of diagnosis

- Diagnosis is used for political and financial purposes and relied upon to make policy concerning the structure and functioning of psychiatric services.
- According to Boyle (1999) psychodiagnosis is neither reliable nor valid (therefore not fit for purpose).

– *Validity* is the degree to which diagnosis represents what it is supposed to and will remain valid and enable reliable prediction even when new information is presented. Diagnosis completely fails to predict prognosis, does not say anything meaningful about cause, nor acts as much of a reliable guide concerning management because of the need to take into account a person's personality and social circumstances. It is therefore scientifically meaningless.

– *Reliability* is the degree to which mental health professionals agree on the diagnosis. This makes diagnosis even more questionable given the arbitrariness of applying diagnostic labels. A good example would be the diagnosis of personality disorder in which a judgement is being made about when personality traits constitute a disorder. Even DSM-IV and ICD-10 are unable to agree on the number of categories for personality disorder, with there being 9 in ICD and 10 in DSM. Van Os (2003) points out that there are 100 different combinations of diagnostic criteria for schizophrenia, which makes the diagnosis of schizophrenia highly questionable in terms of both validity and reliability.

● Reinforces disease explanations of mental disorder at the expense of other perspectives.

The method of assessment and diagnosis

● Arguments similar to those used to challenge positivism and reductionism such as the depersonalising effect of studying 'objects' (*see* the previous chapter).
● By predominantly focusing on the commonalities of experience (the form rather than the content of phenomena), diagnosis ignores human uniqueness.
● It is really a subjective process in the guise of objectivity. Subjective aspects are often unacknowledged or dismissed.

The effects of diagnosis on the individual

● It is an aspect of medicalisation, brought to our attention powerfully by Illich (1995), in which a diagnostic label is given to ordinary experiences and stages of life. Medicalisation, which could also be viewed as pathologising normal psychological distress, may cause harm by creating victims and fostering disabling dependency. It may also divert attention away from social and environmental considerations.
● Diagnosis can be used to label persons in a deliberately negative and harmful way, thus be used as a personal attack that can damage self-esteem. It may also alter a person's sense of identity and social position by becoming an object, or 'the other', with its associated stigma. 'Medicine, like all crusades, creates a new group of outsiders each time it makes a new diagnosis stick' (Illich, 1995, p. 46).
● Diagnosis creates ambiguities around issues of personal responsibility. Having a diagnosis can lead to exemption from responsibility to self and others and can lead to sick-role behaviour. In this situation a person ceases to rely on their own resources and becomes dependent on others. This is an aspect of medicalisation (above).

In summary then, according to Reich, 'diagnosis can turn the fright of chaos into the comfort of the known; the burden of doubt into the pleasure of certainty; the shame of hurting others into the pride of helping them; and the dilemma of moral judgement into the clarity of medical truth' (1999, p. 205). Of course, these sentiments could be uttered as a justification of diagnosis or as a criticism of it.

The person-centred approach to assessment and diagnosis

The person-centred approach is often regarded as antipathetic towards the medical model as practised in psychiatry. Focusing here on assessment and diagnosis only, there is a range of person-centred viewpoints and criticisms that are summarised (in no particular order) as follows:

- The person-centred approach takes a particular stance on the issue of expertise and power. The medical model is viewed as increasing the mystique and power of the helper, which influences the nature of the relationship, creating a power imbalance or even disempowering the patient.
- The assessment process may hinder the development of empathy, as the person-centred approach understands empathy (*see* Chapter 8).
- Assessment and diagnosis can have dehumanising and depersonalising effects. Rogers holds serious reservations about logical positivism and the reductionist tendencies of science, in which persons become objects to be observed in their parts and placed in categories.
- The medical model attempts to *explain* rather than to *understand* and detracts from subjective realities and meaning (more on this in the next section).
- The medical model leads to the tendency to see persons in a fixed state with limited possibilities for change. This contrasts with the person-centred view of persons as being in a continuous process of development towards the fulfilment of innate potential, given the right environment. Rogers writes 'if I accept the other person as something fixed, already diagnosed and classified, already shaped by his past, then I am doing my part to confirm this limited hypothesis. If I accept him as a process of becoming, then I am doing what I can to confirm or make real his potentialities' (1967, p. 55).
- The person-centred approach challenges the legitimacy of mental illness as mental health professionals speak of and view mental illness. It also challenges the over-reliance on disease theories of mental disturbance.
- The medical model is much more focused on what can be objectively described rather than the person-centred emphasis on a person's subjective reality.
- The person-centred approach to therapy is based neither on diagnosis nor on assessment of what is 'wrong' with the patient, but on the potentials within the human organism. The approach aims to provide a facilitative environment characterised by certain conditions, regardless of the diagnosis. In contrast, the medical model involves the provision of diagnosis-specific treatments or interventions.
- The medical model ensures that the 'locus of evaluation' remains firmly in the expert helper. This conflicts with the person-centred approach of facilitating an internal locus of evaluation and taking seriously the patient's frame of reference.

- The directivity of the medical model contrasts with the non-directive attitude of the person-centred approach.

These latter two points deserve, and therefore receive, particular consideration later in this chapter.

Person-centred views range from being strongly opposed to assessment and diagnosis, seeing it as harmful (Shlein refers to diagnosis as 'simply a form of evil' (2002, p. 402)), to those practitioners willing to work with the concepts and process of assessment and diagnosis but translating them into person-centred theory and language. Wilkins believes that 'assessment, although probably not diagnosis in a clinical sense, does have a legitimate place in person-centred therapy' (2005, p. 140). There are also others who wish to develop a person-centred approach to specific disorders, thereby implicitly accepting the legitimacy of medical approaches to diagnosis. Examples include post-traumatic stress disorder (Joseph, 2004; 2005), borderline personality disorder (Bohart, 1990) and 'fragile and dissociated process' (Warner, 2000), although the latter can encompass a range of ICD-10 and DSM-IV categories of disorder.

It should also be noted that assessment is an on-going process. It is an activity that can take place either in or out of conscious awareness. For person-centred practitioners it can include such things as weighing up, for example, relationship potential, or trying to assess how the conditions of congruence, unconditional positive regard and empathy might be received. Within psychiatric settings one of the commonest assessments is of a patient's commitment or motivation to change, especially when considering whether to offer someone therapy. Evaluating people and situations is what human beings do, not just in work contexts or helping situations. It is a process that occupies much of the time and mental activity of mental health professionals.

Rogers actually says very little about diagnosis, although his views can be inferred from his writing. It must also be remembered that what he says is in the context of psychological therapy. In 'Client-Centred Therapy' (1951) Rogers refers to two basic objections. These are concerned with first, the locus of evaluation and second, the issue of power and control. Regarding the latter he points out that 'the long-range social implications are in the direction of the social control of the many by the few' (p. 224). Psychodiagnosis, along with the organisations and systems that rely on it, is clearly seen as having a powerful controlling potential. Rogers is well aware of the social and political implications of diagnosis. However, he doesn't reject the concept of diagnosis. Rather, he sees it differently from the traditional medical model view. One of the most often quoted passages by Rogers regarding diagnosis is as follows:

'In a very meaningful and accurate sense, therapy *is* diagnosis, and this diagnosis is a process which goes on in the experience of the client, rather than in the intellect of the clinician' (1951, p. 223).

He views diagnosis as an evaluative process that takes place within the client in the presence of the therapist, rather than being initiated and imposed on the client by the therapist. In other words, clients evaluate and diagnose themselves, although not necessarily using medical terms. It is from this experiencing within the client that perception and behaviour can change.

Explaining and understanding

A major difference between psychiatry and the person-centred approach is also highlighted by examining the concepts of 'explaining' and 'understanding'. These terms can be clearly delineated to represent two contrasting ways of apprehending mental phenomena. In effect they represent two different paradigms. Explaining refers to the scientist's interpretation of causal laws and reliance on empirical data to elucidate the human psyche as though it can be objectively known. Psychiatry has travelled far along this scientific path. Understanding, however, relates to an interest in how human beings perceive their reality and in the meaning for the individual of their experience. It is not concerned with explanation or definition but in attending to a person's psychological experience *as it is*. Again we are in the realm of subjectivity, rather than the professional's objectivity, where for the helper, empathy is required to understand (which can only ever be partial) how things are for that unique individual. Put simply, psychiatry is often concerned with scientific explanation, whilst the person-centred approach is more interested in the subjective meaning for the patient and in understanding as I have just described it. Thus, two contrasting attitudinal stances are represented – that of empathic engagement with a person versus objectivity and detachment in order to explain the *object* of enquiry. The person-centred approach views understanding and acceptance of experience as more important than explaining it.

It is disregard for personal meaning that contributes to the view that psychiatry, as traditionally practised, is depersonalising. It is perhaps only fair though, to point out that efforts have been made by some psychiatrists to place greater emphasis on the experience of the person. Examples include Meyer's psychobiological model of mental illness (discussed in Chapter 4) and Bracken and Thomas' writing about meaning (2002). So-called Narrative approaches are also attempts to challenge the dominance of the desire to explain mental disorder that fuels the evidence-based culture within psychiatry and medicine generally.

According to Holmes, 'there is no inherent conflict between narrative and evidence-based approaches: understanding the patient's story helps align scientific knowledge with the specific needs and predilections of individual patients' (2000, p. 96). He believes that both approaches can complement each other rather than stand in opposition. Sommerbeck (2003), a person-centred therapist working in a psychiatric hospital in Denmark, holds a similar view when she writes about explaining and understanding being complementary rather than contradictory processes. She uses the analogy of the wave and particle theory in subatomic physics in which photons and electrons can simultaneously and paradoxically be both waves and particles (wave-particle duality), depending on the conditions in which the phenomena are observed. This 'complementarity principle' (proposed by Niels Bohr, one of the founders of quantum mechanics) could also be used to understand the relationship between subjectivity and objectivity, or as a metaphor for the mind–brain inter-relationship as Eisenberg (1986) uses it.

Even if it is possible to pursue both the desire to explain and to understand, the relative weight given to each will directly influence the attitudinal stance towards the patient, communication style and type and quality of listening. Amongst psychiatrists and other mental health professionals there will be enormous variation in emphasis placed on explaining and understanding. However, this will not just be influenced by clinicians' natural inclinations. Of particular influence will be the culture of the mental health setting and the time available for the inter-action. Understanding cannot be rushed. Patients, to tell their story effectively, should not be hurried, and need to have developed sufficient trust that they will be listened to attentively and empathically.

The 'locus of evaluation'

The locus of evaluation was described in Chapter 2 but a recap here may be useful. The locus of evaluation refers to the source of evidence of values and is either internal or external. I have an internal locus of evaluation when I rely on my own judgements and evaluations, and an external one when I rely on the views, opinions and judgements of others as being more valid or important than my own. Clearly then, assessment and diagnosis ensure that the locus of evaluation is external to the patient. The explanatory framework and diagnostic language mental health professionals use take precedence when patients come into contact with mental health services. Patients are expected to learn psychiatry's language and explanations. As a result, many patients come to rely on being told what is wrong with them and on what the diagnosis is, as well as what we, the professionals, believe the treatment should be. In contrast, Rogers (1951) states that 'the client is the only one who has the potentiality of knowing fully the dynamics of his perceptions and his behaviour' (p. 221). Rogers is also concerned with how diagnosis influences the locus of evaluation, stating that '... the very process of psychodiagnosis places the locus of evaluation so definitely in the expert that it may increase any dependent tendencies in the client, and cause him to feel that the responsibility for understanding and improving his situation lies in the hands of another' (1951, p. 223).

The framework for understanding the language psychiatry uses to explain mental disorder is a powerful one. In addition, it concerns me that many patients, even before coming into contact with psychiatric services, have developed poor reliance on their own judgements and interpretation of their experience, believing this to be less valid somehow than that of others. What may then happen is that contact with mental health services further divorces patients from a sense of themselves by imposing 'the truth' as represented by psychiatry. The locus of evaluation becomes even more externalised.

There are many patients who do not present in this way, who actively resist attempts by psychiatry to practise according to the medical model and who challenge diagnostic concepts. As someone with person-centred leanings I notice that I feel more at ease with patients who are able to challenge psychiatric ortho-doxy than with those who are all too ready to be given a diagnosis and told they are ill. I feel distinctly uncomfortable with patients who are extremely eager to know what I think – both what is wrong with them and what to do about it. This is particularly the case for those who have a strong tendency to abdicate personal responsibility and who also wish to place squarely all responsibility with mental health professionals for 'getting it sorted' ('it' being the illness) or 'solving' their difficult circumstances. The medical model and pursuit of diagnosis can reinforce such abdication of responsibility. It is here that the person-centred approach offers an alternative framework for relating to patients and can facilitate the development of an internal locus of evaluation. Unfortunately, I find that a good many patients who are accustomed to mental health services, perhaps having been involved with the service for most of their life, actively resist the person-centred approach to facilitating an internal locus of evaluation. This is an issue of particular significance for those person-centred practitioners working in mental health settings.

The non-directive attitude

The non-directive attitude of the person-centred approach is one of the other major aspects of the approach that stands in stark contrast to the medical model. It was early on in his professional life that Rogers noted the different characteristics of directive and non-directive approaches (1942), and it is implicit in subsequent writing and practice. It later came to be formulated more fully by other practitioners, in part to delineate it from other 'tribes' within the person-centred therapy community who work at different points along a spectrum of non-directivity, corresponding to use of techniques and procedures (Brodley, 2005).

The commitment to the non-directive attitude is fundamentally connected to the belief and trust in a person's tendency to actualise, whilst not forgetting that the right conditions are also necessary for the tendency to move the person forward in the direction of growth. As long as the right environment is provided, characterised by Rogers' six conditions for therapeutic personality change (*see* Chapter 7), there will in effect be no need to tell the client what they need, what they must do, nor what their therapeutic goals must be. The non-directive attitude is firmly embedded in the therapist's practice of the so-called 'core conditions' of congruence, unconditional positive regard and empathy. It is rather unfortunate though, as Tudor and Worrall (2006) point out, that one of the problems of the term 'non-directive' is the tendency to emphasise what the therapist or helper doesn't do.

In addition to the trust in the person's tendency to actualise, another rationale for the non-directive attitude is one based in ethics and values. It concerns a person's right to self-determination. This is a basic respect for a person's autonomy and is a philosophical and ethical stance described by Grant (2002) as 'principled non-directiveness'.

What I think is important to bear in mind when considering the person-centred approach to non-directivity (just as it was important when considering the topic of expertise), is the fact that Rogers was generally writing about it in the context of therapy – originally known as 'non-directive therapy'. However, as described in Chapter 1, the person-centred approach can also be an approach to life and its principles applied outside the therapy context. The questions are: to what extent can or should the non-directive attitude be applied and practised in mental health settings outside counselling and psychotherapy? What level of psychological disturbance, if any, precludes non-directive interventions? When should mental health professionals be directive or paternalistic, if ever? Is detaining or treating someone under the mental health legislation ever justified if the ethical principle of respecting a person's autonomy is to be respected? Does non-directive practice mean not giving advice or asking questions? In responding to these questions I think it is crucial to bear in mind that non-directive practice is not a set of rules, such as never giving advice, but an underlying philosophy. How I practise (my particular behaviours) depends on the patient, the degree and nature of disturbance, and the context. What I do and how directive I am also depends on how I assess someone's 'locus of evaluation'. The more someone is likely to rely on me for advice, or judgements, rather than trusting their own, the less comfortable and inclined I am to give them.

I am only too conscious that much of my practice as a psychiatrist when with patients is highly directive in terms of what I do, particularly when undertaking assessments. I usually have a clear agenda and I direct the process to complete my agenda. In an interview situation with patients I have a structured framework of questions and mental checklist of potential symptoms I want to enquire about. I am also often constructing a management plan in my mind and perhaps formulating a diagnosis. It seems as though the initial interview couldn't be further from the non-directive practice of person-centred therapy. However, I find it helpful to consider the point Brodley makes about non-directivity being an attitude and not a specific behaviour – 'attitudes are *not* defined in terms of behaviours . . . They are defined in terms of intentions, sensibilities, feelings and values' (1999, p. 79). Given this, perhaps despite certain behaviours my role demands of me, it may also be possible to adopt a non-directive attitude to some degree.

It is also important that non-directive practice is not misunderstood as being passive or indifferent, or a way of working that attempts to avoid influencing clients. The person-centred approach is a highly active and disciplined approach because it is about active engagement with clients in the relationship. It is also quite simply impossible for the therapist's or other professional's values and attitudes not to be communicated, however subtly. Facial expression of the listener will convey a lot about their attitude towards what is being communicated. As for subtly influencing content (what the patient talks about and in what way) the quality of listening response is likely to reflect the particular interest of the listener towards the content. In other words, I may be more attentive in my listening to a patient tell her story about her cruel mother than about her weekly ordeal of shopping at the supermarket, conveying that I am more interested in her experience of her mother than of her shopping, thereby influencing what she talks about. But I can be more aware of the way I might influence and of what my ultimate intentions and values are as I listen. Lietaer makes the point that 'it makes little sense to wonder whether a therapist is directive or not. It only makes sense to see *in what way* he or she is directive or task-oriented' (1998, p. 63, original italics).

Another potential misunderstanding is to equate the non-directive attitude with directness, or lack of it, as a style of communication. Being direct, as in being frank and unambiguous in my communication, does not equate with my being directive.

Non-directivity is also not the same as having no goals or no agenda. Speaking about therapy, Brodley says 'all therapies *influence* their clients. The universal goal of therapy is to influence clients towards growth and healing. A therapy *must* influence in order to be effective' (2005, p. 1). In the person-centred approach the general goal is to facilitate constructive personality change and development of characteristics of the 'fully functioning person' (*see* Chapter 2).

Conclusion

I am painfully aware of the number of tensions and inner conflicts I experience in my work as a psychiatrist trying to incorporate person-centred attitudes and values into my work. The psychiatric profession, and the mental health service generally, as I experience them, are generally unquestioning of their medical model methods and their rationale. They tend to follow what Mearns and Cooper describe as the 'A-B-C paradigm' (2005, p. 163), when problem A needs treatment B to achieve outcome C. This is a model that is unable to cope with systemic and holistic principles that sees a multifaceted person in their context with both past and present influences.

It is usually expected that reason and objectivity inform the psychiatric approach, particularly in pursuit of the diagnostic label. I am aware how much this can turn the patient into an object of scientific enquiry who presents a problem to be solved. It is hard to imagine anything more alienating and despair-inducing for a person experiencing mental and emotional distress.

References

American Psychiatric Association (1994) *Diagnostic and Statistical Manual of Mental Disorders* (4th edition). American Psychiatric Association, Washington, DC.

Aquilinia C and Warner J (2004) *A Guide to Psychiatric Examination*. PasTest, Knutsford.

Bohart A (1990) A cognitive client-centred perspective on borderline personality development. In G Lietaer, J Rombauts and R Van Balen (eds) *Client-Centred and Experiential Psychotherapy in the Nineties*. Leuven University Press, Leuven, pp. 599–621.

Boy A (2002) Psychodiagnosis: A person-centred perspective. In D Cain (ed) *Classics in the Person-Centred Approach*. PCCS Books, Ross-on-Wye, pp. 385–396.

Boyle M (1999) Diagnosis. In C Newness, G Holmes and C Dunn (eds) *This is Madness. A critical look at psychiatry and the future of mental health services*. PCCS Books, Ross-on-Wye, pp. 75–90.

Bracken P and Thomas P (2002) Time to move beyond the mind-body split. *British Medical Journal*, **325**: 1433–1434.

Brodley B (1999) About the Nondirective Attitude. *Person-Centred Practice*, **7(2)**: 79–82.

Brodley B (2005) About the Nondirective Attitude. In B Levitt (ed) *Embracing Non-Directivity. Reassessing person-centred theory and practice in the 21st century*. PCCS Books, Ross-on-Wye, pp. 1–4.

Department of Health (2002) *Reforming NHS Financial Flows: Introducing Payment by Results*. Department of Health, London.

Eisenberg L (1986) Mindlessness and Brainlessness in Psychiatry. *British Journal of Psychiatry*, **148**: 497–508.

Freeth R (2007) Political and Philosophical Dimensions of Severe and Enduring Mental Illness. In A Russello (ed) *Severe Mental Illness in Primary Care*. Radcliffe Publishing, Oxford.

Grant B (2002) Principled and Instrumental Nondirectiveness in Person-Centred and Client-Centred Therapy. In D Cain (ed) *Severe Mental Illness in Primary Care*, Ross-on-Wye, pp. 371–377.

Holmes J (2000) Narrative in psychiatry and psychotherapy: the evidence? *Journal of Medical Ethics: Medical Humanities*, **26**: 92–96.

Illich I (1995) *Limits to Medicine. Medical Nemesis: The Expropriation of Health*. Marion Boyars, London.

Joseph S (2004) Client-centred therapy, post-traumatic stress disorder and post-traumatic growth: Theoretical perspectives and practical implications. *Psychology and Psychotherapy: Theory, Research and Practice*, **77**: 101–119.

Joseph S (2005) Understanding post-traumatic stress from the person-centred perspective. In S Joseph and R Worsley (eds) *Person-Centred Psychopathology: A Positive Psychology of Mental Health*. PCCS Books, Ross-on-Wye, pp. 190–201.

Lietaer G (1998) From Non-Directive to Experiential: A Paradigm Unfolding. In B Thorne and E Lambers (eds) *Person-Centred Therapy: A European Perspective*. Sage, London, pp. 62–73.

Mearns D and Cooper M (2005) *Working at Relational Depth in Counselling and Psychotherapy*. Sage, London.

McHugh P and Slavney P (1998) *The Perspectives of Psychiatry*. The Johns Hopkins University Press, Baltimore.

Reich W (1999) Psychiatric diagnosis as an ethical problem. In S Bloch, P Chodoff and S Green (eds) *Psychiatric Ethics* (3rd edition). Oxford University Press, Oxford, pp. 193–224.

Rogers C (1942) *Counselling and Psychotherapy: Newer Concepts in Practice*. Houghton Mifflin, Boston, MA.

Rogers C (1951) *Client-Centred Therapy. Its current practice, implications and theory*. Constable, London.

Rogers C (1967) *On Becoming a Person. A Therapist's View of Psychotherapy*. Constable, London.

Shlein J (2002) Boy's Person-Centred Perspective on Psychodiagnosis: A response. In D Cain (ed) *Classics in the Person-Centred Approach*. PCCS Books, Ross-on-Wye, pp. 400–402.

Sims A (2003) *Symptoms in the Mind. An Introduction to Descriptive Psychopathology*. Saunders, London.

Sommerbeck L (2003) *The Client-Centred Therapist in Psychiatric Contexts. A therapists' guide to the psychiatric landscape and its inhabitants*. PCCS Books, Ross-on-Wye.

Tudor K and Worrall M (2006) *Person-Centred Therapy. A Clinical Philosophy*. Routledge, London.

van Os J (2003) A diagnosis of schizophrenia? In J van Os and P McKenna *Does Schizophrenia Exist?* Maudsley Discussion Paper No 12. Institute of Psychiatry, London, pp. 7–13.

Warner M (2000) Person-Centred Therapy at the Difficult Edge: a Developmentally Based Model of Fragile and Dissociated Process. In D Mearns and B Thorne (eds) *Person-Centred Therapy Today. New Frontiers in Theory and Practice*. Sage, London, pp. 144–171.

Wilkins P (2005) Assessment and 'Diagnosis' in Person-Centred Therapy. In S Joseph and R Worsley (eds) *Person-Centred Psychopathology. A Positive Psychology of Mental Health*. PCCS Books, Ross-on-Wye, pp. 128–145.

World Health Organization (1992) *International Classification of Disease* (10th edition). World Health Organization, Geneva.

Chapter 6

Health, healing or cure?
The person-centred approach
to treatment

'... we are in the work of the helping profession, and the expectation that we solve others' problems is part of our enculturation, our education, and, often, our sense of self-worth'.

(Natiello, 2001, p. 11)

Introduction

Where does the person-centred approach fit into our current mental health service, if at all? This is just one of the questions I shall consider in this chapter, as well as what place there might be for person-centred therapy alongside other forms of psychological therapy. Thinking about these issues leads to a wider consideration of the remit of mental health services today, their goals and under-lying motivations. I continue from the previous chapter my critique of the medical model from a person-centred perspective. I also explore briefly the issue of responsibility and associated issues of freedom and self-determination, since these lie at the heart of the practice of mental health care. The person-centred approach takes these issues very seriously. This leads finally to considering issues of risk and accountability.

I should also point out that this chapter is generally concerned with the person-centred approach to the *issue* (theoretical and philosophical aspects) of treatment rather than person-centred practice itself. Practical applications of the approach are the focus of the next section of this book, beginning in Chapter 7 with a close look at person-centred views on relationship and relating.

Health, healing or cure?

I have a strong memory of an occasion in which a young man in his twenties came to see me in my out-patient clinic. I had known him for a while and he had always struck me as a deeply troubled individual. Indeed, he had been deeply wounded, both by parents who had emotionally abused him and by his school experience in which he was bullied mercilessly. He now seemed to live a rather chaotic existence, never holding down a job for very long and unable to sustain relationships. His sense of self-loathing and lack of purpose contributed to not infrequent admissions following overdoses. He had been diagnosed with an

89

emotionally unstable personality disorder and many of my colleagues and I had come to feel weary whenever he presented in some sort of crisis. We certainly felt frustrated that whatever help we offered seemed to make little difference to his essential feelings of emptiness and low self-esteem. Neither had there been any let up in the frequency with which he harmed himself and took overdoses. Within mental health services this scenario is not rare, even if the details vary. But what was rare (at least for me, and which is why I remember it) was being asked by him so directly and explicitly, as we sat in my clinic, 'Is this condition I have curable?'.

I sometimes muse about conducting an informal survey to find out how my colleagues would respond to this question and to see what the particular styles of response might be, and whether this varies according to profession and training. I don't recall precisely what I replied but I remember that I wanted to convey something of my belief about human beings. I also remember sinking into something close to despair. I think there are several reasons for my emotional reaction to his question. First, I would have to be a pretty uncaring or unfeeling person not to be affected by this young man's plight. Second, I felt a sense of powerlessness because he was desperate for something to take away all his problems, give him a sense of purpose, solve his social and relationship problems, and make him feel good about himself and I was not able to provide this for him. The sort of help he wanted was the 'quick fix' that our society has come so readily to expect and demand. My heart regularly sinks when either I sense or I am clearly told by patients that this is what they want, and what sort of psychiatrist am I if I can't provide it? I become increasingly disheartened by the impossible expectations society and the government place on mental health services and professionals, particularly when responding to what are essentially social issues. Third, I also felt despondent and frustrated because he clearly saw his problems in terms of the medical model. Simply, a diagnosis had been made, so surely we should be able to treat and cure the underlying abnormality? How on earth was I then, in the limited time remaining of our appointment, to attempt to convey something of the concept of personality and personality disorder and steer him away from his notions of correcting some physical disease process with the right pill? Finally, I think what most distressed me was conveying to him my belief that human beings, including him, have an enormous capacity for change and for experiencing healing, whilst also believing that mental health services are generally not able to offer the necessary environment and therapeutic relationships to facilitate this, i.e. an environment characterised by empathic understanding and attitudes of acceptance, for example. I did not share fully my appraisal of mental health services in the interests of preserving whatever hope he may have been clinging to, although it could be argued that I was perpetuating false hope. Indeed, I often wonder how honest I should be about what I regard as the gross limitations and failings of mental health services, certainly in terms of creating healing and therapeutic environments, and particularly for people with disturbed personalities. I think this anecdote demonstrates something of the clash of ideals, expectations and beliefs about what mental health services provide.

Mental health professionals rarely refer to themselves as healers or facilitators of healing. I certainly don't, even though philosophically I am much more at home with these concepts than that of 'problem-solver' or 'fix-it merchant'.

I think my self-concept as a professional helper has a lot to do with the environment in which I work. It seems to be my technical expertise and knowledge that are most demanded, although what is most appreciated by colleagues and patients is hard to tell. Most often it seems I am presented with a problem or dilemma and expected to *prescribe* a solution, often in the form of psychotropic medication, or have the resolution to the dilemma. The language of healing seems such an alien language in today's mental health service. It is not part of the mindset of many (maybe most) of my health care colleagues. Perhaps this is because of its religious overtones, or perhaps because it doesn't sound scientific enough. But I think there is more to it.

Two concepts that come to my mind when thinking about healing are 'wholeness' (incorporating body, mind and spiritual dimensions) and also 'process'. What I think makes them unattractive to mental health professionals and psychiatric services, is that neither concept suggests an endpoint or specific outcome. Healing is not a discrete event but a continuous process. The journey through life until we die could be described as a process towards wholeness, with various factors or relationships facilitating or impeding that process. In contrast, cure implies a specific intervention to a diseased or dysfunctional part of the body or mind. It involves the correction of a disorder of structure or function and a return to normal of something that was abnormal. Cure is not compatible with the multi-dimensional concept of wholeness.

'Recovery' is another concept closely related to healing. Many definitions of recovery exist, one such being:

> '... a person with mental illness can recover even though the illness is not "cured". ... [Recovery] is a way of living a satisfying, hopeful, and contributing life even with the limitations caused by illness. Recovery involves the development of new meaning and purpose in one's life as one grows beyond the catastrophic effects of mental illness' (Anthony, 1993, p. 15).

The recovery model is trying to establish a place within mental health services, particularly through the National Institute for Mental Health in England (NIMHE). It is a model based on values-based practice rather than evidence-based practice, an approach that is usually user-led, which focuses on a person's strengths rather than deficits, and which aspires to genuine empowerment. However, it faces an uphill struggle to become established in the current culture, given the dominance of the scientific, biomedical paradigm and mental health policy driven by the desire for measurable outcomes, cost-effectiveness and efficiency. Despite the rhetoric of mental health policy sounding as though it supports concepts of wholeness and recovery, it is the modernist, biomedical paradigm of evidence-based practice it really champions because this represents all that is rational and scientific. Furthermore, cure rather than recovery speaks the language of measurable outcomes so desired by politicians and managers.

Notions of a person's innate capacity to recover and to heal are also sometimes resisted. A good example of resistance amongst psychiatrists to ideas of recovery as an inner process is the commonly held view that people with personality disorder don't recover because the disorder just 'burns itself out'!

What enthusiasts of the concepts of recovery and healing probably have in common are certain ideas about what constitutes mental health. In forming a view of what mental health consists of, patients' subjective realities – which include social, cultural and religious dimensions – are taken seriously, rather than placing an emphasis on the supposedly objectively assessed mental state. Mental health can exist regardless of the presence or not of mental illness. Placing health and illness on a continuum is another common way of viewing health. What many definitions of mental health have in common are notions of, for example, the ability to survive pain and disappointment, having a positive sense of well-being, positive self-image and identity and ability to learn and develop as life situations change. The ability to make and sustain intimate personal relationships has also been considered a key ingredient of mental health, as well as having a sense of personal autonomy and social justice. One of the descriptions I like is the view that:

'to be healthy is not to correspond with some fixed norm, but to make the most of one's life in whatever circumstances one finds oneself, including those which in terms of some fixed norms may seem severely impaired or unhealthy' (Boyd, 2000, p. 14).

Yet in many mental health settings such a view of mental health tends to be rare in my experience.

The person-centred approach speaks the language of recovery, healing and wholeness, as well as appreciating the above concept of mental health that is concerned with potentialities, rather than deficiencies.

What drives mental health policy?

The predominant goal of mental health services is to treat the diseased part and correct the deficiency, rather than to enable a process of healing and wholeness. But what is wrong with this? Isn't this a reasonable and sensible goal and perhaps the only viable one in a tax-funded public institution, such as the NHS, that inevitably has limited resources? (I suspect that managers of private insurance-based mental health services would recognise even less the concepts of healing and recovery, preferring those of treatment and cure.) Yet whilst it is only right to have serious debate about the goals, priorities and remit of services, I think it is shocking that a health care culture has developed that not only struggles to provide healing, therapeutic environments and relationships, but which can actually be harmful, to both patients and mental health professionals alike.

The culture I find myself working in is one dominated by a 'rigorous pursuit of efficiency and cost-effectiveness' (DH, 1998, p. 64). This of course is largely political speak for saving money. In themselves, efficiency and cost-effectiveness are not unreasonable aspirations and personally I dislike inefficiency, disorganisation and waste, flaws in the NHS which it seems justifiable to remedy. Yet the manner in which and the degree to which these goals have been pursued since the Labour government came to power in 1997, and since embarking upon a massive programme of reform of mental health services, have led to a culture that is obsessed with targets and the erosion of personal qualities and values. Thorne puts this is the strongest possible terms. To him our culture (including that of health care settings) 'has increasingly fallen victim to the savage onslaught of an economic philosophy based upon depersonalising concepts of efficiency and cost-effectiveness' (1997, p. 163).

This obsession leads to the provision of treatments, interventions and activities whose outcomes, in terms of symptom reduction or behavioural change, can be measured, rather than to an interest in some inner shift of feeling and thinking that may not be objectively demonstrable. If the results can be measured then there is a chance that the intervention or treatment can be said to be proven and therefore described as evidence-based. It is predominantly these goals that motivate politicians and managers as services are reorganised. The human values of co-operation and trust are further undermined by the creation of a system based on a market economy that uses competition to 'drive up standards'. The primary goal has now become that of managing resources rather than caring for people in their time of need and vulnerability.

For the health system to work according to the goals of government and management, treatment approaches need to be standardised and it needs to be possible to decide easily which groups of patients should be given which treatment and by whom. Categorisation of patients according to diagnosis is important here too. If it becomes possible to measure the activity of mental health professionals and specific outcomes of treatments then the government will also be able to apply their proposed funding arrangements in mental health as well as the rest of the NHS – 'Payment by Results' (DH, 2002) – the potential consequences of which appal me. Diagnosis will become even more relied upon to determine treatment. The medical model of assessment, diagnosis and treatment is therefore perfectly suited to the type of mental health system (and health system generally) that the current government wishes to develop.

In contrast to providing quick cures for well-defined problems, providing environments and services that facilitate healing and recovery require more resources and financial investment. Mental health professionals must be allowed to have the time to develop relationships with their patients, rather than to process them through the system on care pathway conveyor belts. However, it is not simply a matter of resources, the resource here being time. A mental health service that aspires to do more than treat symptoms or fix the immediate problem, requires a fundamental change in the culture and attitudes that underlie debates about costs and allocation of time and other resources. At present though, I see little enthusiasm for giving serious attention to these more fundamental issues, fundamental, that is, if we want a mental health service in which therapeutic relationships can develop and be maintained, and where healing can occur.

Psychiatric versus person-centred approaches to treatment

As noted in the previous chapter, treatment is the final step in the medical model sequence of assessment, diagnosis and treatment. The question 'What is the treatment?' depends for its answer on asking 'What is the diagnosis?'. This is the first observation I would like to make about treatment approaches within psychiatric settings, which I summarise as follows:

- It is diagnosis-driven, and the more disorder-specific the treatment the better.
- When the diagnosis is not clear, or even if it is, the treatment usually aims to reduce or eradicate symptoms.

- The more quantifiable, and therefore measurable, the outcome the better. For treatments to be acceptable to politicians and managers they need to be evidence-based. The randomised-controlled trial is the gold standard when it comes to evidence-based research, with the underlying value being scientific objectivity.
- There is a culture within mental health settings that *doing* something *to* the patient, i.e. applying an intervention, is usually necessary and a good thing.
- Treatment approaches try to rely on explanatory theories about what has caused the disorder. Commonly applied are disease theories, with the biochemical imbalance theory being the most relied upon.

The following statement, whilst referring to psychotherapy programmes and therapeutic techniques, demonstrates many of the above observations:

> 'Increased neuroscientific knowledge will help us to help the brains of our patients to devise and make use of sometimes complex and sometimes simple mental strategies to cope with weaknesses in their brain function, whether these are caused by genetic vulnerability, developmental assault or a unique combination of the two' (Fonagy, 2004, p. 358).

Treatment approaches within mental health settings are often an eclectic mixture of psychological and pharmacological interventions, according to what resources are available. In other words, there is an over-riding need to be pragmatic at the expense of ideology and theoretical consistency. Unfortunately, mixtures of interventions can make it very difficult to know which is the most and which the least helpful. In these instances clinical judgements and intuition are often relied upon, although increasing moves to standardise care will limit reliance on subjective judgements. The National Institute for Clinical Excellence (NICE) endeavours to issue guidelines for specific disorders, with guidance based on the evidence-based research available. Needless to say, psychotropic medication and cognitive-behavioural therapy (CBT) feature prominently as treatments of choice. Both attempt to reduce and eradicate symptoms, which in the case of CBT, is generally to correct faulty thinking or learn coping strategies. Both attempt to produce measurable outcomes and can be applied relatively easily in a structured or manualised fashion making them suitable for quantitative research.

From what I have already discussed about the person-centred approach from previous chapters, it should not be hard to see just how little in common the approach has with current psychiatric practice. In fact, even to call the person-centred approach a treatment will be to many person-centred practitioners, including myself, anathema. It certainly does not aspire to cure people; 'indeed the concept of cure is quite foreign to the [person-centred] approach we have been considering' (Rogers, 1951, p. 230). It will therefore be hard for the person-centred approach to sit alongside traditional psychiatric treatments. In the same passage, Rogers describes the person-centred approach more as 'a point of view which might in basic ways be applicable to all individuals, even though it might not resolve all the problems or provide all the help which a particular individual needs', whilst also acknowledging that some people may need hospital care or medication. He does not therefore position the person-centred approach or therapy as an alternative to compete with traditional treatments when those treatments seem necessary.

Some of the specific conflicts with medical model treatments include the fact that the person-centred approach does not rely on diagnosis. Person-centred principles apply whatever category of disturbance a person is described as having. Indeed, in the field of psychotherapy, Bozarth goes so far as to describe particular methods of treatment for particular dysfunctions as the 'specificity myth' (1998, p. 164). Arguments opposing diagnosis were outlined in the previous chapter, many reflecting what is regarded as its depersonalising tendencies and lack of honouring a person's uniqueness. Another difference is the anti-reductionist stance of the person-centred approach, in attempting to meet the whole person rather than treat the abnormal part or remove the symptom. In fact, Bryant-Jefferies makes the point that it may not be helpful to remove the difficult and painful symptoms and that these symptoms might actually be an aspect of the healing process. He says, 'Perhaps the inner experiencing needs to be allowed to exist in awareness with the client being offered warm acceptance and empathic sensitivity to what is becoming present' (Bryant-Jefferies, 2005, p. 178). I certainly think it is tragic when patients receive the message that they are acceptable, and understandable, only when their symptoms are removed. In other words, whilst psychiatry is more likely to view symptoms as negative and needing eradicating, the person-centred approach aims not to attach such value judgements and is more interested in the patient's subjective experiences and what these experiences might mean.

Regarding goals then, even though it is true that the person-centred approach will not be primarily focused on symptoms (at least in terms of trying to remove them), it is not the case that the approach does not have any goals. Broadly, the goal of the person-centred approach (or perhaps more accurately, the goal of the person-centred therapist or helper) is to provide the *conditions*, through *relationship*, to enable constructive personality change, to empower a person to use the resources within them and to facilitate their tendency towards growth and the characteristics Rogers describes as experienced by the 'fully functioning person'.

In pursuing this general goal, however, the person-centred approach is much more interested in the *process* rather than specific *outcomes* or final destination, and hence is not measurable for the purposes of quantitative research. This will not of course appeal to managers. The fully functioning person (described in Chapter 2) describes a person in the process of becoming all that he or she is able to become. There is no final point of arrival because human beings are constantly in a process of development. However, it is interesting to question whether person-centred practice is necessarily resistant to quantitative research. Certainly the pressure is on the person-centred community to show that it isn't totally resistant, lest the approach be ignored even more.

Another significant contrast highlighted in the previous chapter is the much greater emphasis the person-centred approach places on a person's subjective experience, and this experience being understood for its own sake and for what it might mean to that individual, rather than the professional or therapist seeking an explanation or interpretation of it. This of course leads to criticisms that the person-centred approach is unscientific, with its lack of interest in defining persons and their mental states objectively.

Psychiatric approaches also generally consist of *doing to* the patient, in contrast to the person-centred emphasis on *being alongside* and, as Rogers puts it, 'freeing him for normal growth and development' (1942, p. 29). This by no means implies that being alongside (or being with) someone is passive, as sadly it tends to be perceived. Worse is the way this activity is given such low status, evidenced by the regularity with which health professionals refer to 'just' being with, or 'just' listening. The power of relationship and connecting with people is often ignored or not recognised, in the desperate need to ensure that one is looking busy and doing things *for* patients, particularly if that activity can be recorded and measured. It is the particular attention to the relationship that is unique to the person-centred approach, even if in our attention to that relationship we are unfairly dismissed as 'not doing much'. In fact it is often in the 'not doing' that the skill lies. Sometimes being busy with tasks is as much about fulfilling our own needs as it is about helping the patient, and it may actually disempower the patient, along with using approaches that rely on demonstrating the helper's expertise over and above facilitating the patient's inner expert.

Finally, although this analysis is by no means exhaustive, the person-centred approach to helping can be described as a developmental approach, although not in the sense of working through 'stages of development'. Rather, it is interested in human potential and working to strengths rather than deficiencies or deficits, which is the more common focus of psychiatry. Furthermore, it is more optimistic about the inherent potential of human beings to develop and our capacity to overcome and cope with difficulties. However, to free this potential requires great trust in the presence and power of human beings' innate potential, and perhaps one of the most significant contrasts between psychiatry and the person-centred approach is the willingness to trust that this potential can be released. Many mental health professionals are often more ready to be cynical than optimistic, and for mental health professionals to trust in a person's tendency to actualise will require a great deal of courage and a willingness not to succumb to the more prevalent pessimistic attitudes and the climate of cynicism that mental health settings often generate.

Any place for person-centred therapy?

It would be a mark of courage for managers of mental health services to decide to employ person-centred therapists and counsellors, given what I have said about the current culture and what drives mental health policy. It would require an ethical commitment to a set of values and philosophy that could not be easily depicted by a spreadsheet or described in managerial jargon. That these values and ideals are not generally recognised at political or managerial levels, or by influential leaders of the various mental health professions, partly explains why it is rare to find person-centred therapists working within secondary care, either on their own or as part of a psychological therapies or other team.

Within secondary mental health services person-centred therapy is usually not regarded as a credible approach relative to other forms of psychological therapy, according to criteria of effectiveness such as the randomised-controlled trial of evidence-based research. It generally cannot compete with, for example, biological psychiatry (the use of medication) and CBT because of, for example, its different goals, such as symptom reduction or removal. It is also quite common for psychiatrists to hold disparaging attitudes towards person-centred therapy and counselling. It certainly does not help when eminent psychiatrists such as

Professor Sir David Goldberg suggest that counsellors whose approach is non-directive be retrained to provide the 'appropriate skills' so that patients are not being deprived of adequate intervention (Goldberg and Gournay, 1997, p. 15). For these authors there is no room for non-directive approaches. They are generally regarded as not evidence-based and not having the efficacy of medication and cognitive behavioural interventions, even though some research has demonstrated that non-directive counselling approaches are as effective as CBT in reducing depressive symptoms within primary care (King, Sibbald, Ward *et al*, 2000). The person-centred approach, as a non-directive approach, is also often regarded as passive and benign. This is a misunderstanding that does considerable damage to the credibility of the approach, and is, unfortunately, a view shared by many psychiatrists.

According to 'Treatment Choice in Psychological Therapies and Counselling' (DH, 2001) CBT is the form of therapy that achieves first prize in terms of its evidence base. It is considered first-line therapy for many disorders such as depression, anxiety disorders, post-traumatic stress disorder and eating disorders. In the more recent document 'Organising and Delivering Psychological Therapies' (DH, 2004), it is clear that the agenda is to provide services according to which form of therapy works best for which diagnosis. Roth and Fonagy's highly acclaimed book 'What Works for Whom?: A Critical Review of Psychotherapy Research' (2004) is another good example of the importance attached to diagnosis when evaluating evidence in the field of psychological therapy.

What also seems to be required of psychological therapy services is the ability to provide evidence of their effectiveness, efficiency and quality (DH, 2004) as part of both clinical governance and performance management. So-called 'performance indicators' are increasingly demanded. This has led to the development in the UK of standardised systems to measure outcomes, with the leading system being the Clinical Outcomes for Routine Evaluation (CORE) system. CORE is an increasingly popular evaluation and audit tool that enables benchmarking of services. Given what I have said previously about the person-centred approach neither lending itself to objective measurement nor defining outcomes in terms of medical model notions of treatment and symptom reduction, it is not hard to see why person-centred therapy and counselling often find themselves dismissed or ignored within NHS secondary care.

There are other issues which lead to the general perception that person-centred therapy is not suitable for secondary care mental health settings. The person-centred approach is more often thought of as a form of counselling rather than psychotherapy, with counselling historically having more of a place in primary rather than secondary care. Furthermore, it is often thought that it is only suitable for the so-called 'worried well' or those with less severe psychopathology, and certainly not those with severe mental illness. This raises two issues. The first involves the commonly held distinction between psychotherapy and counselling. The second issue concerns the suitability, or not, of psychological therapy for more severe psychological disturbance.

Taking the issue of counselling versus psychotherapy first, it is a confusing picture. 'Treatment Choice in Psychological Therapies and Counselling' (DH, 2001), uses Psychological Therapy as a generic term for two different activities, whilst acknowledging some blurring in the middle of a continuum, with counselling at one end and psychotherapy at the other. However, what this continuum represents is not made clear, but it probably represents the commonly held distinction which is that psychotherapy is a more in-depth activity that may occur over a longer time period and that psychotherapists have undergone lengthier and/or more intense training. The implication here is that psychotherapy is a superior activity to counselling because more expertise is possessed by the more highly trained therapist (psychotherapy training generally calls for more hours training than that for counselling). This certainly tends to be the view of the status and hierarchy-conscious medical profession.

This document also suggests that counselling and psychotherapy are different activities (perhaps two continua are needed) because 'Different forms of counselling emphasise the individual's resources rather than psychopathology ... There is emphasis on mental health promotion rather than "treating disorders"' (DH, 2001, p. 8). To me this implies that counselling is thought of as different from psychotherapy, the latter being concerned with the more serious matter of treating disorders, rather than simply enabling people to 'develop a greater sense of well being' (p. 8). In summary, differences are as follows:

- the diagnosis and the severity of the client/patient group
- the nature of the activity, with psychotherapy tending to be seen as the medical treatment
- the setting, with counselling mostly occurring within primary care
- the vested professional and personal interests of many who prefer to regard themselves as psychotherapists for reasons of status and, in the private arena, financial gain.

What does the person-centred approach have to say to all this? It may come as little surprise that the person-centred approach regards counselling and psychotherapy as interchangeable terms, seeing no essential difference in the activity of providing a therapeutic relationship and environment regardless of whether one chooses to describe oneself as a counsellor or psychotherapist. Neither the diagnosis, nor the severity of disturbance makes a person unsuitable for person-centred therapy, provided psychological contact is established. 'Contact' is the first of Rogers' six conditions for therapeutic change. Furthermore, even if psychological contact is impaired, the person-centred approach has developed a method known as 'Pre-Therapy' for reaching contact-impaired clients (Prouty, Van Werde, Pörtner, 2002) as Chapter 9 explores. The only limitations of offering person-centred therapy are those imposed by the individual therapist's competence and confidence. There is also now plenty of evidence of person-centred therapy being practised with people with deeper psychological disturbance (Joseph and Worsley, 2005). Finally, the jostling for power and status that the 'is it counselling or is it psychotherapy' debate often involves, could be seen as evidence of the vested self-interests of professionals, the consequences of which are ultimately harmful to the therapy profession and the patients and clients it seeks to serve.

Returning then, to the potential place for person-centred therapy alongside other therapies within mental health settings, I believe it might have a chance of becoming more recognised were mental health services to heed the call in an article in the 'British Journal of Psychiatry' (Guthrie, 2000) for a new research paradigm. In this paradigm, psychotherapy is not researched according to what type of therapy works for which diagnosis, but according to patient characteristics such as 'personal compatibility' or readiness and motivation. Patient expectations and the degree of hope (the patient's and the therapist's) might be other characteristics. This certainly seems to reflect other significant research in the form of an extensive meta-analysis showing that therapy effectiveness depends to a large extent on the quality of the therapeutic relationship (30% variance) and extra-therapeutic variables – internal and external resources of the client (40% variance). In other words, 70% of outcome variance has nothing to do with the type of therapy (Lambert, 1992). Other research has led to a search for the 'common factors' for positive outcome in psychotherapy (Hubble, Duncan and Miller, 1999). Likewise, Jeremy Holmes, a well-known psychiatrist and psycho-therapist in the UK, suggests that 'psychotherapy research and practice must move beyond "brand names" of different therapies to an emphasis on common factors, active ingredients, specific skills, and psychotherapy integration' (Holmes, 2002, p. 288). It is also interesting to note that Roth and Fonagy, whose extensive research into 'what works for whom', state in their book of the same title, that 'In general "brand names" rarely predict outcomes and in direct comparisons most studies show a broad equivalence between therapies' (1996, p. 28). In other words, after all the outcome research conducted over the years, no one model or technique can claim superiority over any other. This, in my view, endorses the importance of future research along the lines Holmes suggests. Despite common factors such as the relationship between patient/client and therapist being difficult to research, such research does exist. Norcross (2002) has edited an important book that examines empirical research into understanding the thera-peutic relationship.

It is of course also imperative that users of services make their voice heard in influencing the shape of psychological therapy services and ensuring that they are both fully informed and have genuine choice as to whether, for example, they want a therapist who practises primarily in a relational way or a therapist who sees themselves as more of an expert in the use of techniques and whose style and practice are more about teaching the client skills.

Without relational therapies and their values I believe the mental health system currently being created will become more dehumanised and will continue to create countless casualties amongst both patients and staff. Without a genuine recognition of the importance of the relationship in therapy (i.e. more than just a theoretical acknowledgement), psychological therapies will continue to become more 'manualised' and the therapist will eventually be replaced by a computer programme. Indeed, such programmes already exist, and have been successfully used, along with self-help books, and they surely have their place. I simply wish it wasn't called therapy because for me psychological therapy fundamentally requires relationship.

Freedom: a right, a capacity and a responsibility

It is not possible to move on from the subjects of treatment and the functioning of mental health services without considering the issues of freedom and responsi-bility. Along with the subjects of autonomy and self-determination, with which they interweave, these are profound philosophical subjects in their own right. However, considering them in the context of psychiatry and NHS mental health services presents a complex web of issues I can only hope to superficially untangle a little here.

It is these issues that, in my day-to-day clinical practice as a psychiatrist, cause me some of my most troubling dilemmas and uncertainties. Issues of freedom, responsibility and self-determination cut to the heart of what I believe and value about human beings, as well as how an ethical mental health service should function and the wider issue of how society takes care of vulnerable people. This leads also to a consideration of our attitudes towards risk. It is also fair to say that person-centred therapists and other advocates of the person-centred approach are likely to find themselves in considerable conflict with the prevailing culture within psychiatric settings.

The person-centred approach places extremely high value on individual freedom and as a libertarian society we value the idea that we are free agents. However, valuing a concept and allowing it to inform our practice and behaviour are two different things. As a general observation, person-centred practitioners are much more likely to honour a person's freedom in practice as well as in theory, compared to mental health professionals. The latter are often concerned that without intervention and a degree of coercion, he or she might be held accountable and blamed if there are negative consequences. I shall say more on this later.

In thinking about and trying to understand the concept of freedom, three dimensions of it have emerged for me. The first is to consider the issue that human beings have a *right* to make their own decisions and choices, even if they are choices we might consider bizarre or even irrational. This is what is meant by having our autonomy respected and it is one of the main ethical principles health professionals are expected to abide by. The right of every adult to make his or her own decisions is recognised in the new Mental Capacity Act 2005. For some person-centred therapists, the ethical right to self-determination is the very foundation of their non-directive practice (Grant, 2005; Witty, 2005).

A second dimension that often raises itself within psychiatry is considering whether a person has the *capacity* to make decisions and should therefore be *allowed* to act freely without intervention. (Within medicine, 'capacity' refers to the ability of a person to make decisions about treatment and a legal definition has now been proposed, included in the Mental Capacity Act.) Here again, the person-centred approach can contribute powerfully to this debate. It would take issue with the degree to which mental health professionals often intervene to restrict a person's freedom by detaining them using mental health act legislation, or coercing patients into making decisions professionals believe are in the patient's best interests, viewing such use of power and control as damaging, as well as wrong. The person-centred view is also one that is more likely to see the existence of a capacity within people to make decisions. Schmid puts this clearly when he says 'Anyone who subscribes to the person-centred approach ... is convinced of and thus has faith in the fact that every human being possesses the capacity to shape his or her life and that the main objective of every form of aid should be to support this capacity, that is to promote human freedom and autonomy' (1998, pp. 38–39). This person-centred view is not one I have heard very often within psychiatric settings, and certainly not the theory that this capacity and tendency for self-determination are manifestations of the actualising tendency.

For person-centred practitioners, the practical consequence of a belief in the capacity for self-determination is to provide the conditions through a particular quality of relationship and relating and by adopting the non-directive attitude. Yet, as I have discussed, the medical model is in conflict with the non-directive attitude. Psychiatry is slow to recognise the expertise and resourcefulness within patients or that patients might know what is best for themselves. It is also worth noting that when there is doubt about a patient's capacity, one of five key principles of the Mental Capacity Act previously mentioned, is the *presumption* of capacity. It must be assumed that patients have capacity unless proved otherwise. However, whilst this is upheld in general medicine for physical illness, when it comes to psychiatry and mental illness the rules seem to change, with that presumption no longer applying.

Where the debate becomes particularly difficult is when and how capacity for self-determination and making decisions are affected in the context of mental disturbance. It is assumed all too readily that decision-making capacity is impaired in people with mental disorder, leading to intervention against their will and therefore discrimination against people with mental disorder. Indeed, it has been argued that in this respect, current mental health legislation is discriminatory (Szmukler and Holloway, 1998), and lacks respect for the autonomy of mentally ill people (Doyal and Sheather, 2005). It is discriminatory that an adult with capacity is allowed to refuse treatment for a physical disorder but not for a mental disorder (Bellhouse, Holland, Clare *et al*, 2001). It may well be that some forms of mental disturbance impair capacity, especially when thought processes and cognition are grossly disrupted. In my view though, the assumption of impaired capacity is made too readily for people who come into contact with the mental health system and by virtue of receiving a psychiatric diagnosis, and is used as a justification for intervening forcibly or coercing people into accepting treatments.

I want to consider a third aspect of freedom that also has profound implications for mental health practice. This is the concept of responsibility. According to Tudor and Worrall (2006), Rogers, along with other American existentialists, 'overlooked or chose to ignore the European recognition that if we are free we are also responsible, and that, in an isolated and meaning-free life that ends necessarily in death, responsibility is, potentially, as distressing as the idea of freedom is exhilarating' (p. 30).

Freedom and responsibility then, are intertwined. Yet it is significant how much, within society generally, the one (freedom) is desired whilst the other (responsibility) is rejected. Within mental health settings the issue of responsibility is particularly significant because mental disorder and diagnosis are often viewed as exempting people from responsibility for their behaviours and from societal obligations. Many patients are happy to hand over responsibility to professionals, wanting us to take sole responsibility for their mental well-being, being happy to be passive recipients of care.

The issues of dependency and sick-role behaviours are some of the most difficult to respond to. Unfortunately, I think there is regularly a willingness on the part of mental health professionals to avoid these difficult issues. Too often the psychiatric system colludes with patients who want to hand over responsibility. There are probably many and varied reasons for this. Challenging dependency and sick-role behaviours requires sensitivity and can be a lengthy process, requiring patience, especially if it is the system that has fostered dependency in patients over many years in the first place, which is often the case.

It also requires the whole system to be giving the same message and too often different parts of the system and different professionals give conflicting messages. It requires mental health professionals not to get into what Johnstone describes as 'The Rescue Game' (2000). How many of us are natural rescuers? How many of us are aware that we are, and are willing to have supervision to examine the ways in which we are tempted to rescue people by relieving them of responsibility and thereby fostering dependency? Perhaps lack of effective supervision within mental health settings is another reason why it is all too common for mental health professionals either actively to remove responsibility from patients or passively to allow them to abdicate it, without necessarily being aware that this is happening. We need to learn how to curb our paternalistic and rescuing tendencies, when they occur, that is, if we believe that patients have the right and capacity to make their own decisions and decide their own goals.

Does mental disturbance legitimise some degree of passivity? Does it depend on the type of disturbance and the personality of the individual? Can we be responsible for some things and not others? These are difficult yet important questions that need regular discussion (and therefore space and time for such discussion) within mental health settings, and must be allowed to inform our practice.

One thing I experience regularly is the 'double-bind' of much of psychiatric practice. For example, the system fosters dependency because we are expected to take responsibility for patients with mental disorder. This comes through government policy and mental health legislation as well as, often, from patients themselves. At the same time the system and mental health professionals (especially psychiatrists) are often condemned for being controlling and misusing their power. In addition, patients who have become dependent are often those whom mental health professionals find the most challenging and may dislike working with. This issue of being blamed for whatever one does or doesn't do is one of the most wearying and stressful to deal with in my work. I could do well, however, to regularly remind myself of one of the components of ethical practice in 'The Capable Practitioner' in which mental health professionals are to 'encourage self-determination and freedom of choice' (The Sainsbury Centre for Mental Health, 2001, p. 10), which of course captures the spirit and philosophy of the person-centred approach. In addition, I need to develop coping mechanisms to deal with being or feeling condemned when that occurs.

Finally, I want to return to the idea of self-determination as a capacity, but to look at it more broadly than as a medical term that focuses on intellect, cognitive processes and functioning. I also want to consider something of Rogers' viewpoint on self-determination in terms of the debate about free will versus determinism.

So-called 'hard determinists' regard all events as caused or determined by antecedent conditions such that we cannot be responsible for our decisions, thinking and actions. In this camp are scientists such as Francis Crick who believe that there is a 'neural correlate' for 'free will' and that the seat of the 'will' is at or near the anterior cingulate sulcus in the brain (1994). For biological psychiatrists it is only a matter of time (or at least it is theoretically possible) before we understand the scientific laws that control all our brain processes – all our thoughts and decisions. Computer analogies of cognitive processes or the conditioning behavioural theories of BF Skinner, also suggests that we are more causally determined than we are free agents.

Often this debate is represented as a continuum, with defenders of free will (libertarians) at one end and hard determinists at the other. This means of course that there is a grey area in between where it is possible to believe in both causal determinism and the notion of free will, a somewhat paradoxical position which, according to Merry (1995), was the one that Rogers occupied. The scientist part of Rogers believed that human beings are influenced by their genetic make-up and their environment (conditions of worth being powerful environmental influences). However, his attraction to existentialist theories led to his commitment to the existence of free will. Merry draws our attention to part of a dialogue Rogers held with Skinner in which Rogers says:

'I am in thorough agreement with Dr Skinner that, viewed from an external, scientific, objective perspective, man is determined by genetic and cultural influences. I have also said that in an entirely different dimension, such things as freedom and choice are extremely real' (Kirschenbaum and Henderson, 1990, p. 139).

For me it is by no means clear how much to hold people responsible for their choices and behaviours when in the context of mental disorder such as mental illness or personality disturbance. I do believe though that in mental health settings we should assume patients have much more responsibility (with its associated freedom) than in fact we do.

One of the difficulties in dealing with the issue of responsibility is the way we think of and talk about it, i.e. language can be misleading. Is responsibility a 'thing' that can be given and removed or passed around? Or is it a capacity or a process? When we 'give' responsibility to or 'remove' responsibility from people it is not the case that we are removing their innate capacity to take responsibility. Rather, we are influencing their opportunities to exercise their capacity to take responsibility. We are giving or removing opportunity. We develop our capacities (for all sorts of things) through the opportunities we are given or denied. So the more opportunity I am given to take responsibility, the more likely I am to develop my capacities to take responsibility. The point I am trying to make then, is that by denying people responsibility and freedom to make decisions concerning their behaviours (this being the tendency of current mental health practice largely in response to the public protection agenda, fear of litigation, but also perhaps because we underestimate peoples' capacity to take responsibility), they are being denied the opportunity to exercise and develop their capacities. Our capacity to take responsibility and make decisions as free-thinking adults is profoundly shaped by the behaviours of others around us and cultural assumptions about what human beings have a capacity to do or not do. The person-centred approach aims to increase peoples' sense of freedom and responsibility and to do this it is important to assume that the capacity exists within the individual and has the potential to be exercised given facilitative conditions.

Risk and accountability

Unfortunately, not only would an advocate of the person-centred approach lament the health care culture of obsessive concern with efficiency, measurable activities and outcomes, the dominance of evidence-based practice at the expense of values-based practice, and cost-saving measures over and above providing healing and safe environments; he or she must painfully acknowledge that the health service is also a culture of fear, mistrust and free-floating anxiety. I am not referring here to patients but to NHS employees, and it is not hard to imagine something of how this affects the quality of our care of patients.

Within mental health services this springs in part from the current government's preoccupation with public protection in which 'risk avoidance and public safety have become the new watchwords' (Laurance, 2003, p. xiii), at the expense of civil liberties and providing a therapeutic service. In his book, Laurance explores how mental health services are being driven by fear and have become more coercive and controlling to avoid risk. The recently proposed mental health legislation provides ample evidence of this. This practice of attempting to control risk is also clearly highlighted by Julia Neuberger (2005) in her book exploring the political, social and moral decline in the UK. Professionals have become wary of an 'inquiry culture' following high-profile homicides in the late 1990s. This fear of being blamed when things go wrong inevitably leads to more risk-avoidant and back-covering behaviours. I regularly find myself in the situation of wanting to encourage 'positive risk-taking' by not taking responsibility for a patient's risk-taking behaviour and not intervening when patients are threatening to kill themselves, when I believe they have and should be encouraged to take responsibility for their behaviours. At the same time the level of fear and anxiety within and around me amongst colleagues, as well as the threat of condemnation that I would be acting either irresponsibly or uncaringly is a pressure hard to resist. The message is always to play safe, to fear the coroner's court or inquiry panel, do a risk assessment, then do another, and to record verbatim every conversation in the notes. All the while anger and frustration may mount and it becomes hard not to act punitively towards the patient who has now perhaps had their freedom removed and will as a result not have had an opportunity to manage their own risks and learn to take responsibility for their own well-being.

Our society's fear and 'crisis of trust' as described by O'Neill in her book 'A Question of Trust' has also created a culture of micromanagement, of excessive regulation, where increasing concern about accountability is experienced as *distorting the proper aims of professional practice* and indeed as damaging professional pride and integrity' (2002, p. 50, original italics). She also suggests that making people and institutions more accountable may increase suspicion, which in turn increases surveillance and fuels paranoia. Thorne expresses similar sentiments when he writes about the '... death-dealing culture of accountability and appraisal where the basic assumption is that no-body is really trustworthy and where everyone has to be monitored and given incentives if they are to do a good job' (1998, p. 57). The NHS is as much infected with these concerns as other institutions, private and public. In contrast, according to Rogers 'the person-centred approach is built on a basic trust in the person' (1990/1986, p. 136). However, he also recognises that 'this is perhaps its sharpest point of difference from most of the institutions in our culture' (*ibid*).

My dismay is the way this health care culture of fear and mistrust affects our relationships with patients and with colleagues. We may lose the ability to relate openly and transparently, to see the constructive potential in people, to be forgiving and to be creative. Our relationships become strained, we close down, we are not able to listen and we watch our backs. We lose our sense of well-being and may become sick, decide to work part-time or retire early. The culture of mental health services as I experience it is toxic, psychologically disturbed and dysfunctional. It is often a wonder to me that it can call itself a mental health service.

References

Anthony W (1993) Recovery from mental illness: The guiding vision of the mental health service system in the 1990s. *Psychosocial Rehabilitation Journal,* **16(4)**: 11–23.

Bellhouse J, Holland A, Clare I and Gunn M (2001) Decision-making capacity in adults: Its assessment in clinical practice. *Advances in Psychiatric Treatment,* **7**: 294–301.

Boyd K (2000) Disease, illness, sickness, health, healing and wholeness: exploring some elusive concepts. *Journal of Medical Ethics: Medical Humanities,* **26**: 9–17.

Bozarth J (1998) *Person-Centred Therapy: A Revolutionary Paradigm.* PCCS Books, Ross-on-Wye.

Bryant-Jefferies R (2005) *Responding to a Serious Mental Health Problem. Person-Centred Dialogues.* Radcliffe Publishing, Oxford.

Crick F (1994) *The Astonishing Hypothesis. The Scientific Search for the Soul.* Simon and Schuster, London.

Department of Health (1998) *Modernising Mental Health Services. Safe, sound and supportive.* Department of Health, London.

Department of Health (2001) *Treatment Choice in Psychological Therapies and Counselling. Evidence Based Clinical Practice Guidelines.* Department of Health, London.

Department of Health (2002) *Reforming NHS Financial Flows: Introducing Payment by Results.* Department of Health, London.

Department of Health (2004) *Organising and Delivering Psychological Therapies.* Department of Health, London.

Doyal L and Sheather J (2005) Mental health legislation should respect decision making capacity. *British Medical Journal,* **331**: 1467–1469.

Fonagy P (2004) Psychotherapy meets neuroscience. A more focused future for psychotherapy research. *Psychiatric Bulletin,* **28**: 357–359.

Goldberg D and Gournay K (1997) *The General Practitioner, The Psychiatrist and the Burden of Mental Health Care.* Maudsley Discussion Paper No 1. Institute of Psychiatry, London.

Grant B (2005) Taking Only What is Given: Self-determination and empathy in non-directive client-centred therapy. In B Levitt (ed) *Embracing Non-directivity. Reassessing person-centred theory and practice for the 21st century.* PCCS Books, Ross-on-Wye, pp. 248–260.

Guthrie E (2000) Psychotherapy for patients with complex disorders and chronic symptoms. The need for a new research paradigm. *British Journal of Psychiatry,* **177**: 131–137.

Holmes J (2002) All you need is cognitive behaviour therapy? *British Medical Journal,* **324**: 288–290.

Hubble M, Duncan B and Miller S (1999) *The Heart and Soul of Change: What Works in Therapy.* American Psychological Association, Washington, DC.

Johnstone L (2000) *Users and Abusers of Psychiatry. A Critical Look at Traditional Psychiatry Practice* (2nd edition). Brunner-Routledge, London.

Joseph S and Worsley R (eds) (2005) *Person-Centred Psychopathology: A Positive Psychology of Mental Health.* PCCS Books, Ross-on-Wye.

King M, Sibbald B, Ward E, Bower P, Lloyd M, Gabbay M and Byford S (2000) Randomised controlled trial of non-directive counselling, cognitive-behaviour therapy and usual general practitioner care in the management of depression as well as mixed anxiety and depression in primary care. *Health Technology Assessment,* **4(19)**: 1–83.

Kirschenbaum H and Henderson V (eds) (1990) *Carl Rogers: Dialogues.* Constable, London.

Lambert M (1992) Implications of outcome research for psychotherapy integration. In J Norcross and M Goldfield (eds) *Handbook of Psychotherapy Integration.* Basic Books, New York, pp. 94–129.

Laurance J (2003) *Pure Madness. How Fear Drives the Mental Health System.* Routledge, London.

Merry T (1995) *Invitation to Person Centred Psychology.* Whurr Publishers, London.

Natiello P (2001) *The Person-Centred Approach: A passionate presence.* PCCS Books, Ross-on-Wye.

Neuberger J (2005) *The Moral State We're In. A Manifesto for a 21st Century Society.* Harper Collins, London.

Norcross J (ed) (2002) *Psychotherapy Relationships That Work: Therapists' Contributions and Responsiveness to Patients.* Oxford University Press, Oxford.

O'Neill O (2002) *A Question of Trust.* Cambridge University Press, Cambridge.

Prouty G, Van Werde D and Pörtner M (2002) *Pre-Therapy. Reaching contact-impaired clients.* PCCS Books, Ross-on-Wye.

Rogers C (1942) *Counselling and Psychotherapy: Newer Concepts in Practice.* Houghton Mifflin, Boston, MA.

Rogers C (1951) *Client-Centred Therapy. Its current practice, implications and theory.* Constable, London.

Rogers C (1990) A Client-centred/Person-centred Approach to Therapy. In H Kirschenbaum and V Land Henderson (eds) *The Carl Rogers Reader.* Constable, London, pp. 135–52. (Original work published 1986)

Roth A and Fonagy P (1996 – 1st edition; 2004 – 2nd edition) *What Works for Whom?: A Critical Review of Psychotherapy Research.* Guilford Press, New York.

Schmid P (1998) 'On Becoming a *Person*-Centred Approach': A Person-Centred Understanding of the Person. In B Thorne and E Lambers (eds) *Person-Centred Therapy. A European Perspective.* Sage, London, pp. 38–52.

Szmukler G and Holloway F (1998) Mental health legislation is now a harmful anachronism. *Psychiatric Bulletin,* **22**: 662–665.

The Sainsbury Centre for Mental Health (2001) *The Capable Practitioner. A framework and list of the practitioner capabilities required to implement The National Service Framework for Mental Health.* The Sainsbury Centre for Mental Health, London.

Thorne B (1997) Counselling and Psychotherapy: The Sickness and the Prognosis. In S Palmer and V Varma (eds) *The Future of Counselling and Psychotherapy.* Sage Publications, London, pp. 153–166.

Thorne B (1998) *Person-centred Counselling and Christian Spirituality. The Secular and the Holy.* Whurr Publishers, London.

Tudor K and Worrall M (2006) *Person-Centred Therapy. A Clinical Philosophy.* Routledge, London.

Witty M (2005) Non-directiveness and the Problem of Influence. In B Levitt (ed) *Embracing Non-directivity. Reassessing person-centred theory and practice for the 21st century.* PCCS Books, Ross-on-Wye, pp. 228–247.

Section Two:

Practical applications of the person-centred approach

Chapter 7

The healing power of relationship

'Especially in our present age, when science and fact and proof are held in topmost esteem, it is unfashionable, to say the least, for a professional person to assert the moving quality and therapeutic potency of something one cannot put one's finger on, which is not subject to precise description, item-isation, quantification, analysis, or even to verification by one or more of the five senses.'

(Perlman, 1979, p. 22)

Introduction

What I find so extraordinary about the above words, referring as they do to helping relationships, is how relevant and accurate they are over twenty-five years from when they were written. Within health care settings the scientific, biomedical paradigm continues to hold sway, as does the preference for object-ivity and measurement. In my view, the quality of relationships with patients, whilst almost universally acknowledged as important, is in practice often ignored, neglected or simply overshadowed by other pressing concerns.

This chapter turns the spotlight on the helping relationship, asserting that not only is attending to it important, but that to do so is in fact vital if we are genuinely interested in the mental health and healing of those entrusted to our care. Rather than simply presenting an idealised vision of healing relationships though, particularly from a person-centred perspective, I think it is also impor-tant to recognise the real barriers to developing such relationships and the influence of the health care environment and context. I shall therefore spend some time exploring how current mental health services and policies place considerable constraints on developing relationships of any depth and quality. I shall also look at some of the current types and characteristics of relationship and the emphasis on developing communication skills rather than developing our selves and our attitudes.

This chapter also serves to introduce Rogers' theory of therapy which consists of the six conditions he identifies as necessary for psychological growth, otherwise referred to as 'constructive personality change'. Of these conditions, congruence, unconditional positive regard and empathy will be discussed in Chapter 8.

It is important to point out that what Rogers has to say about therapeutic relationships is not limited to the therapy relationship. Likewise, this chapter concerns therapeutic relationships with mental health professionals who may or may not be therapists and in which the context may or may not be therapy. Too often, in my view, therapeutic relationships are regarded as the sole province of psychotherapists and psychologists, even though it may be the case that therapy can provide the conditions in which the therapeutic relationship is particularly potent and transformational. According to Rogers 'the therapeutic relationship is seen as a heightening of the constructive qualities which often exist in part in other relationships, and an extension through time of qualities which in other relationships tend at best to be momentary' (1957, p. 101). Sometimes it is the momentary smile or non-judgemental word of kindness that can bring about transformation. Sometimes only moments are needed.

The significance of relationship

I think quite often mental health professionals do not realise the profound impact, positive and negative, of their relationship with, or manner of relating to, patients. Perhaps it is only through being on the receiving end of a helping relationship, or knowing someone who is, that one realises how powerful this experience can be. I shall never forget the smile and gentle enquiry as to how I was from a nurse at a day hospital I attended during a period of time away from medical school with depression. This followed a harrowing few days in which my levels of despair had intensified and I had not attended. I had expected expressions of disapproval for not having informed the day hospital I would not be attending, as well as negative judgements for having contemplated ending my life. To receive that brief expression of genuine concern and kindness whilst feeling so emotionally fragile and fearful of judgement was priceless in its simplicity. It had a very profound impact upon me.

I would like to recount another experience that has played no small part in shaping my attitudes towards therapeutic relationship and relating and which contributed to making my training to be a person-centred therapist somewhat inevitable. This experience occurred several years later, having completed my year as a junior house officer and now embarked upon psychiatric training. I was in my first six month post as a psychiatric senior house officer (SHO) and had been asked to assess a man on a general medical ward who had taken an overdose. This was a routine referral, although by no means routine for me, being an inexperienced SHO approaching the ward with a degree of trepidation. This was immediately exacerbated by the ward sister wishing me good luck and saying, 'He won't speak to you ... He won't talk to anyone and says it is a waste of time asking a doctor to visit'. Now this would not have been so bad if the overdose had been impulsive, not life threatening and quickly regretted by the patient. This would mean I need not worry too much if I were to leave the ward without having conducted a formal assessment for the possibility of an underlying mental illness or risk of further overdoses in the near future. The risk would clearly be low. Unfortunately, this was a well-planned suicide attempt. This man had intended to die, having left notes for people and put his affairs in order. He had expressed regret that the overdose wasn't 'successful' and had been hostile to the general medical team and to the nurses on the ward, presumably angry that his attempt had been scuppered and that he was receiving medical attention he did not want. These were the bare facts given to me before I approached his bed wondering what on earth I was to do if he refused to talk to me and I was none the wiser as to whether he had a serious mental illness, had continuing suicidal intent and perhaps even needed to be detained for his own safety. Could I let him walk out of hospital not knowing anything further about him and worrying or suspecting that he might be at high risk of further suicide attempts? The stakes seemed high to achieve some sort of psychiatric assessment.

What I remember after introducing myself was saying something that acknowledged he didn't want to talk to me, to which he agreed in a hostile way that I was indeed wasting my time. However, there must have been something about my manner or even initial empathic understanding of his desire not to talk that somehow connected with him. He did spontaneously start to talk. I, in turn, abandoned my previous agenda of conducting a standard psychiatric assessment and just listened to whatever he wanted to say. In the end he had told me enough for me to be satisfied that he didn't have a mental illness, nor did he have any immediate plans for trying to end his life again, although his sense of seeing little point in living meant that he couldn't exclude the possibility in the future. I was happy for him to be discharged from hospital without any psychiatric follow-up and wished him well. The next day he turned up unexpectedly at my place of work (in a different part of town from the hospital), and asked for a few minutes of my time. He apologised for his initial hostility towards me in the hospital and he wanted to tell me that he had done some thinking and what his plans were. For now he was going to try to work through some of the problems that had led him to attempt suicide. He thanked me for listening to him in the hospital and said that in future when he found himself in difficulty and needing to think things through, he would imagine himself talking to me.

In my work since, both as a psychiatrist and as a counsellor, I have not received any greater confirmation of the power of listening, empathic understanding and acceptance than this. It was not specific communication skills that made the difference, but, I believe, a way of relating therapeutically that may well have facilitated the beginning of a healing process. As much as my role as a psychiatrist still requires me to gather information, conduct a mental state examination and assess for the presence of mental illness, I have not forgotten that it is also worth attempting to do so in a way that I hope may be experienced by the patient as therapeutic. Of course, how much I achieve this depends on the situation, the patient, the time available, and my attitudes and readiness to listen, which often depend on my energy and stress levels.

These two experiences in particular have taught me a lot about the importance of therapeutic relating and a way of being in a relationship that may be experienced as healing. On both occasions I believe something significant was experienced between two people. Something was communicated by the person in the helper role that was experienced as powerfully enabling to the other. This 'something' could only be experienced through relationship, through a connection being made.

Relationship is so fundamental to being human. It has been described as 'the primary medium of human life' (Barrett-Lennard, 2005, p. xi) and as the 'mover and shaker and propulsive force in human life' (Perlman, 1979, p. 23). We are relational beings who need to bond with other human beings. Our healthy emotional and personality development depends on the existence of strong, nurturing bonds as infants and children. Our need for relationship is part of our 'hard wiring', not just to *bond* but also to *communicate* and *interact* (Mearns and Cooper, 2005). Mearns and Cooper offer a concise review of research and the academic literature on the importance of relationship from a developmental perspective, including Rogers' hypothesis of the infant's need for positive regard (described in Chapter 2).

It is therefore no surprise that a good proportion of people who come into contact with mental health services or psychotherapy and counselling services, are those who have experienced various disturbances in relationships, either in their past or in their present. My own observation and experience lead me to agree with Mearns and Cooper that much psychological disturbance is associated with a lack of healthy and nurturing relational experiences, or loneliness.

As most of us know, loneliness is much less concerned with physically being on one's own and more to do with lack of connection, of not feeling understood and heard by those with whom we are in relationship. Barrett-Lennard (2005), who regards loneliness as endemic in our culture, offers a helpful analysis of many forms of loneliness, including 'estrangement from oneself' (such as not knowing who we are) and 'interpersonal loneliness' (lack of connections with others and sense of belonging) and 'hunger for community'. This leads him to see the urgent need for relational healing, not just on an individual level but within families, communities and societies.

I am now uncomfortably aware that some mental health professionals may respond to such an analysis of loneliness, the value of relationship and need for relational healing by wondering what this has to do with mental health services. Is this not society's problem that should therefore be tackled on a societal level? Or if it is part of our task as mental health professionals to respond to the relational needs of our patients, how can we do so with any measure of effectiveness given the current ethos and culture within mental health services? It is to this question I shall now turn.

Can mental health services offer healing relationships?

Even to talk about healing relationships within mental health settings is to risk being confronted with puzzled expressions at best and cynical dismissal at worst.

Whether services and mental health professionals offer healing relationships depends upon two related issues. First, are such relationships a desirable and legitimate goal of mental health services? Second, if they are, is it possible to offer or cultivate them?

To many of us, it is being able to offer healing relationships that has brought us into the mental health professions. Perhaps our belief in its importance has been forged through our own experiences of mental suffering and being offered such a relationship ourselves. Caring through relationship and attending to its quality is for many of us our *raison d'être*. Yet it seems to me as though this is an increasingly minority position given many of the issues I have highlighted so far in this book such as the dominance of the medical model, the focus on psychopathology, concern for treating the disease and other such reductionist approaches. A deep valuing of healing relationships is becoming harder to find amongst colleagues, and certainly amongst managers and politicians, given what is generally considered the more important quest for objectivity, categorising the patient by diagnosis, placing them on the correct care pathway and referring them to the 'appropriate' team within the service to achieve the desired measurable outcome. Services are being developed in which patients are 'processed' through the system to allow each intervention and outcome to be measured and costed.

The overarching goal of mental health services (and the NHS in general) is to 'deliver health care' and to 'provide a service' in the most evidence-based and cost-effective way possible. The culture of mental health services and policy making is infused with the business ethic of delivering the product, hitting the targets and managing resources. Providing healing relationships is not, it seems, part of this overall goal and cannot compete with the task of achieving these other organisational objectives, currently of recouping large debts. In this respect health services have come to reflect the values of society in general, in which attending to the quality of our relationships, and knowing how to nurture them, are given short shrift and cannot compete with, for example, materialistic values and economic concerns. Thorne points out:

> 'The increasing drivenness of many people, and the ravages of competitiveness and technological innovation, mean that quick "cures" and a rapid return to functional efficiency are frequently demanded by clients who have neither the time nor the inclination to seek below the surface for the cause of their ills' (2002, p. 7).

Could it be that mental health services collude with societal values in not giving time or attaching importance to enabling relationships to unfold and develop as natural processes, and failing to connect beneath layers of superficiality? Yet, if mental health professionals cannot recognise the profound despair of loneliness in their patients, understand the yearning for honest relating with the person behind the protective mask, and be in relationship with patients in a way that enables them to feel understood and heard at depth, is this not a tragedy for our society? Perhaps it is the absence of healing relationships within mental health services that fuels further the levels of despair and loneliness within society. For it is surely an extra and bitter blow not to experience understanding or sensitive relating from those from whom one might most expect it.

Even if mental health professionals do value and strive to cultivate healing relationships with their patients, as a core philosophical and caring ideal, there are nevertheless considerable constraints to putting this ideal into practice. The structure of our jobs, our working environments and the way we are required to work are major ones. Some of my regular struggles include the volume of work, its nature and unpredictability, being required to juggle many tasks and different roles, having to prioritise constantly, and in general simply survive the pressure and stresses of the work and the workplace. Bureaucracy is another well-recognised barrier to attending to relationships. The amount of documentation required has reached extraordinary proportions, much of it in the interests of risk management, risk assessment, or to put it less politely, back-covering. Constant overload of information – guidance, policies, directives, memoranda, etc. – also interferes with the cultivation of relationships.

Levels of general fear and mistrust within mental health services (as described in Chapter 6), poor relationships with colleagues, badly managed and poorly functioning teams, lack of consideration for the general well-being of staff, all contribute to low morale which will have a direct effect on quality of care and relating. If health care organisations do not become what Barrett-Lennard describes as 'human-relations systems, ones in which the relationships and well-being of members have become a natural and self-perpetuating priority' (2005,

p. 125), there is little hope of being able to be helpful let alone cultivate deeply healing relationships with patients.

What we have now are organisations that see themselves as trying to provide a 'functional' service, the 'delivery' of which will be 'performance managed'. This translates as mental health professionals and teams being required to focus on their 'functions' and tasks. In other words, emphasis is placed on the activities we perform. Referring to the medical profession, Roy describes how 'the emphasis is shifting to aspects of "performance" that lay out what a doctor should *do* to be a good doctor rather than what a doctor *is* to be a good doctor' (2004, p. 5, original italics). This is a culture that is problem- and activity-based, in which mental health professionals have to demonstrate their capabilities, of which 36 are identified in 'The Capable Practitioner' (The Sainsbury Centre for Mental Health, 2001), with many of these subdivided and many added depending upon the type of mental health setting. In a health care culture of demonstrating competencies and 'doing' for or to others, preferably performing activities and tasks that are visible and measurable, relationship can easily be, and often is, overlooked or viewed in the most superficial terms.

Types of relationships within mental health services

The term 'therapeutic relationship' is a very general term and can be conceptualised in many different ways. This section aims to explore some of the common ways of thinking about the therapeutic relationship within mental health settings and some of the characteristics that are commonly associated with it. To begin with, I am grateful to Tudor (1999) for making the distinction between relationship and relating, the latter being an activity (a verb rather than the noun of relationship). Very often I think mental health professionals talk about the relationship whilst really referring to a set of helper behaviours or ways of relating.

I think there is a tendency to generalise when we talk about the therapeutic relationship. Therefore, it is worth highlighting just how many different ways it is viewed, both within and between professions. For example, psychiatrists vary hugely in how they regard relationship and in how much emphasis they place on it theoretically, philosophically and in clinical practice. Whether a relationship is viewed as something to be 'managed' or seen as something mysterious with remarkable healing and growth-promoting properties, impacts hugely on the connections we may or may not attempt to make in that relationship. Relationships with patients also vary enormously according to their context, including the particular problems or psychopathology that have brought a person into contact with psychiatric services, whether patients are in hospital or at home, voluntary or detained, what the patient's expectations are and a host of other variables.

I think there is also a tendency to view the therapeutic relationship as solely the province of therapists or psychologists, reflected by the fact that most literature on the therapeutic relationship comes from the therapy professions. However, there is a long academic tradition within mental health nursing exploring the concept of 'caring' and the nature of the 'nurse–patient relationship'. Reynolds describes the therapeutic relationship as the 'crux of clinical nursing' (2003, p. 139). Other key figures from within mental health nursing have written powerfully on the importance of relationship, particularly focusing on aspects of caring, such as Barker (2000) and Watkins (2001). Some authors go further. Stickley and Freshwater, for instance, consider the art of loving in the nursing relationship (2002).

Nevertheless, these days much focus tends to be on the 'skills' involved in relationship. This is certainly the case in the medical profession, with the emphasis on communication skills and styles of relating. Doctors are encouraged to review these skills regularly as part of continuing professional development (British Medical Association, 2003) and they are increasingly taught in a formal way at medical school. The emphasis is usually on tasks and learning techniques such as how to gather information or how to run the consultation (Gask and Usherwood, 2002). Other key tasks include how to give non-verbal encouragement or frame questions. Indeed, there are now comprehensive lists of skills for doctors to learn and develop such as the Calgary–Cambridge Guides, which list some 71 skills to be used as required (Silverman, Kurtz and Draper, 2005). Communication skills education also tends to focus on particular scenarios such as how to break bad news or deal with difficult situations.

What I think is regrettable is that the emphasis on developing communication skills is increasingly motivated by an awareness of how failures of communication often lie behind complaints and litigation (British Medical Association, 2003), rather than because they may be helpful in their own right. Another rationale for learning communication skills is that 'patients are more likely to adhere to treatment and to follow advice' (Maguire and Pitceathly, 2002, p. 697).

Sladden (2005) recommends learning various 'psycho skills' to put in one's 'treatment toolbox'. Thus, not only are skills something to perform, they are also embedded within the medical model. Skills are applied as part of relating to the patient as part of the treatment, just as the mechanic selects his tool to fix the broken part of the machine.

The emphasis on skills for most non-medical NHS staff is also reflected in, for example, the 'Knowledge and Skills Framework' (DH, 2004). Here knowledge and skills are applied to provide 'a single, consistent, comprehensive and explicit framework on which to base review and development for all staff' (p. 3), the demonstration of which is clearly linked to career and pay progression.

What is very common in my experience of health care settings is the notion of relationship as something to *use* as a tool in order to solve problems or to facilitate client development. The relationship is viewed as a means to an end. There are a few points I wish to make about this. First, the relationship is often referred to when it is really a set of behavioural skills that are being described. Egan's (2004) popular 'The Skilled Helper' model exemplifies this, with the focus on what and how to *do* in the relationship rather than how to *be* in the relationship. Egan's approach places the emphasis on the problem. Indeed, he believes that overly focusing on the relationship is a distraction from the goal of helping the client manage the problem.

Second, a similar point is described by Hirschhorn (1997) who distinguishes between the *role* and the *person*, identifying a tension between them, and suggesting that modern organisations favour the role.

Third, whilst the helper is applying a set of skills or using the relationship to achieve a goal, which often only they decide, they are directing a process and not trusting the resourcefulness of the patient to both determine the goal and work towards it in their own way. This clearly contrasts with the non-directive attitude of the person-centred approach I describe in Chapter 5. An analogy is the difference between the helper being a travelling companion and a travel agent (Peck and Norman, 1999). I contend that many mental health professionals are good travel agents but very poor travelling companions, by which I mean we are good at telling patients in what direction they should head and how to get there, rather than travelling with them.

The role of the mental health professional, with the emphasis on their skills, leads me next to consider another way of viewing the relationship, one that places more emphasis on the role of the patient or client. The 'therapeutic alliance', sometimes known as the 'working alliance', is the term and concept I want to focus on next. This is a term with psychoanalytic origins and it is a concept frequently used by the counselling and psychotherapy professions as well as within mental health settings. It captures the notion of collaboration and it has been described as the 'quality and strength of the collaborative relationship between client and therapist in therapy' (Hovarth and Bedi, 2002, p. 41).

Three components of the therapeutic alliance have been identified and described by Bordin (1994). These components are bonds, goals and tasks. The quality of the alliance relates to the level of agreement between helper and client about goals and tasks, and this is mediated by the attitudes and styles of relating (bonds) between helper and client. I think it is the notion of bonds that would find most resonance with the person-centred approach.

Although the therapeutic alliance refers to notions of collaboration, it does not automatically imply a sense of equality or mutuality in the relationship, mutuality being an important person-centred concept referring to reciprocity in relationships. The presence or absence of equality and mutuality with patients will depend upon the context and the values and philosophy of the mental health professional. It will depend on the helper's attitudes towards power, embodiment of authority and reliance on their expertise, level of trust in the patient's inner resources and belief in their right and capacity to self-determination. Within mental health settings, a common view of the therapeutic alliance is as a tool to achieve the professional's pre-determined goals and using the authority of the professional to aid compliance. In other words, the therapeutic alliance can be *used* directively and manipulatively, which runs counter to the person-centred approach as previously explored in Chapter 3 on power. Or is it the case that when manipulation or coercion is occurring, the term therapeutic alliance no longer applies?

The therapeutic alliance is in fact just one of five types of relationship identified and described by Clarkson in her book 'The Therapeutic Relationship' (2003). Other types of relationship are the 'transference/counter-transference relationship', the 'developmentally-needed or reparative relationship', the 'person-to-person or real relationship' (closest to the person-centred conceptualisation of relationship) and the 'transpersonal relationship'. Whilst Clarkson describes all these relationships in the context of therapy, their characteristics can certainly exist outside therapy. In mental health settings the concept of the transference/counter-transference relationship receives some attention, although less so these days as biological psychiatry has come to dominate thinking and practice.

Related to the concept of transference is the idea of 'professional distance'. Within the therapy professions, particularly psychodynamic orientations, such distance may be deliberately created to encourage the development of transference

(transference being the term used to describe the phenomenon of transfer-
ring emotions and attitudes from one person to another, e.g. from a parent to
the therapist, largely unconsciously). According to Sigmund Freud (1953) the
physician needs to be opaque and like a mirror to the patient, showing nothing
but what is shown to him or her. Professional distance here is concerned with the
therapist deliberately withholding personal material from the patient. However,
whilst mental health professionals are often cautious about self-disclosure and
may be taught to reveal little of themselves, it is usually to avoid criticisms of
over-involvement rather than to foster transference.

Keeping an 'appropriate' professional distance (whatever this is) can refer to
another idea, namely, that of emotional detachment. I can think of two reasons
for this. First, psychiatrists, at least, are taught to cultivate objectivity, the suggestion being that becoming emotionally involved with patients distorts the ability
to be objective and therefore interferes with making sound clinical judgements.
The second reason is simply to survive the job emotionally. Doctors learn to
become emotionally detached during their training, both as an instinctive coping
mechanism and through the advice of medical colleagues and formal teaching.
According to Gask, 'Junior doctors cope with the demands of all medical specialties by learning how to be emotionally detached. Psychiatry is no exception'
(2004, p. 74). My own experience concurs with this, although when I find myself
feeling detached, it is not in response to advice (I am not sure how much one can
do this as an act of will, although supervision might regulate levels of emotional
involvement), but because detachment seems to be an automatic self-protective
response to overwhelming demands. Whilst emotional detachment is perhaps
sometimes an inevitable and understandable, although regrettable, consequence
of working in mental health settings, and other settings in an under-resourced
NHS, I object to the notion of keeping a professional distance as though this is the
mark of a competent professional. It is a style of relating and emotional dis-
engagement that I think can be powerfully rejecting and alienating for patients
when they encounter it in mental health professionals. It is contrary to the
person-centred commitment to personal involvement and to offering the conditions for constructive personality change. I shall consider these conditions in the
next section.

The person-centred approach to relationship

Although the person-centred approach to relationship is most often described in
the context of therapy, it can apply to a wide range of health care and non-health
care settings. It is fundamentally a philosophy of human beings and relationship
that manifests as a 'way of being' and 'which fits any situation in which *growth* –
of a person, a group, or a community – is part of the goal' (Rogers, 1980, p. xvii).
At the core of this philosophy of relationship are the experiencing and communication of certain *attitudes*. Writing about psychotherapy Rogers puts this as follows:

'Contrary to the opinion of a great many psychotherapists, I have long held
that it is not the technical skill or training of the therapist that determines his
success – not, for example, his skilful dream interpretations, his sensitive
reflections of feeling, his handling of the transference, his subtle use of
positive reinforcement. Instead, I believe it is the presence of certain *attitudes*

in the therapist, which are communicated to, and perceived by, his client, that effect success in psychotherapy' (1990/1959, p. 10, original italics).

It is the emphasis on the attitudes of the helper or therapist that is so distinctive and radical, rather than the more prevalent concern in health care settings with the demonstration and practice of certain listening techniques and communication skills. In other words, the primary emphasis for the person-centred practitioner is not what they do but who they are and the attitudes they embody in the relationship.

This is of course a major challenge to the more expert-orientated approaches in which helpers are not only required to demonstrate their knowledge and skills, but it is these skills that are regarded as the agents of change. According to Bozarth, the theory of person-centred healing relationships 'militates against the use of techniques. Techniques are generally problem-centred and therapist-driven rather than trust-centred and person-driven. They are generally laden in one way or another with the expertise of the therapist' (1998, p. 121). The tendency of the person-centred approach to reject the reliance on techniques and specific interventions (such as giving advice, or using cognitive-behavioural strategies) is, therefore, related to two aspects of the approach. First, it is not primarily a problem-solving approach. Rather, the emphasis is on facilitating the innate potential and resources within individuals towards growth and development, rather than the helper identifying deficits that have to be corrected. The second aspect concerns the non-directive attitude of the person-centred approach, where trust is placed in the patient's innate tendency to actualise under certain specified facilitative conditions or attitudes. The rejection of the use of techniques is not some kind of rule to be followed slavishly, but is, rather, the consequence of trust in the individual that if they are in relationship with a helper who embodies certain attitudes, they will be able to move forward in a constructive fashion.

However, it is perhaps worth mentioning that within the person-centred therapy community there is debate about the use of techniques and interventions. It is these differences of opinion that have contributed to the development of several 'tribes' within the person-centred family, these tribes being therapies that have departed somewhat from Rogers' original (or 'classical') approach. Or have they? This is the debate: whether such techniques that might be used in, say, person-centred art therapy or Eugene Gendlin's 'Focusing' (1978), represent a form of directivity that ceases to place trust in the individual and the actualising tendency and which relies on the expertise of the therapist. Personally, I like what Rogers says on the subject: '. . . the techniques of the various therapies are relatively unimportant except to the extent that they serve as channels for fulfilling one of the conditions' (1957, p 102). In other words, if unconditional positive regard and empathy are communicated through techniques then they are acceptable, but this is difficult to do without a weakening of the non-directive attitude.

For an NHS mental health professional it is impossible to avoid the plain fact that the whole of mental health practice is predicated on interventions, the use of expert advice, communication skills or behavioural strategies. This is part of the job description for most of us, i.e., to assume the role of expert and to intervene appropriately. Nowhere does it specify the experiencing and communication of certain attitudes and I suspect that many mental health professionals might struggle to articulate what their attitudes are towards human beings and relationship. We learn how to behave towards patients in a certain way but not to think about why we behave the way we do. How much of the way we are with patients is grounded in a clearly articulated philosophy of relationship and relating? The person-centred approach, in contrast, is an integration of belief, philosophy and practice. This is why it is distressing for person-centred practitioners to witness how the approach is frequently misunderstood to consist of, for example, simply the application of empathy as a technique or behavioural response.

Even though in my practice as a psychiatrist I am often being directive and, for example, giving my opinion and advice as expected and requested of me, I can still at least be mindful of my attitudes whilst doing so, and try to be aware of how my interventions are perceived by patients. I also try to be aware that the effect of my advice giving or interventions on patients will vary greatly depending on their locus of evaluation, i.e., their ability to rely on their own judgements, and not on external authorities, as to what to think, decide or do. Thus, I am much less hesitant about giving advice if I trust that that individual is able to weigh it up and ultimately decide what to do for themselves. For those patients who have a very poorly developed self-reliance and who have learnt to be passive when experiencing authority figures, I am conscious that I will be perpetuating their dependence on others and lack of trust in their own judgements by being directive and giving advice. Unfortunately, this way of working (e.g. advice-giving) seems impossible to avoid in the current climate of mental health services and what is generally expected and requested of mental health professionals. Much of current psychiatric practice colludes with patients deferring to expert advice and opinion and trusting less their own experiencing and judgements. Nevertheless, we can attempt to limit our use of techniques, interventions and advice giving and attempt to embody more a way of being that patients may experience as healing and facilitative.

The person-centred approach then, is more than the establishment of a therapeutic alliance. It can be described as fundamentally a relational approach, i.e., one that uniquely emphasises relationship. It is about making connections with people. As Natiello puts it (2001, p. 25):

> 'The quality of the relationship goes far beyond what we know, what we do, and how we do it. It is really about *who we are* – the spiritual, emotional, attitudinal characteristics that we embody as persons, our ability to make a deep connection, to tolerate intimacy, and to offer a climate of safety'.

It can involve interpersonal encounters that transcend whatever else patients may experience or use, such as medication. It views relationship as the primary source of healing which goes beyond the cure of problems or eradication of symptoms. The person-centred approach is one that can facilitate what Mearns and Cooper term 'relational depth': 'a state of profound contact and engagement between two people' (2005, p. xii). Only in relationship can a person be understood and understood in a way that has the potential to heal. I believe that the person-centred approach offers a special quality of understanding.

Rogers' theory of therapy

Having made some general points about the person-centred approach to relationship, I now want to turn to, arguably, the most significant contribution to the therapy professions and helping relationships in general. This is Rogers' theory of therapy. However, I want to reiterate that although Rogers mainly presents his theory in the context of a therapy relationship, it applies to relationships in general where the goal is one of growth and healing.

The person-centred approach to therapeutic and healing relationships consists of the presence of six conditions and this formulation, according to Thorne, 'remains as radical and disturbing as it did 40 years ago' (2003, p. 36). Whilst much attention is usually given to the three conditions of congruence, un-conditional positive regard and empathy, it is all six that, together, are considered 'necessary and sufficient' for psychological change and growth. I shall return to the idea of necessary and sufficient later, but for now these conditions are simply stated as follows:

'1. That two persons are in *contact*.
 2. That the first person, whom we shall term the client, is in a state of *incongruence*, being *vulnerable* or *anxious*.
 3. That the second person, whom we shall term the therapist, is *congruent* in the *relationship*.
 4. That the therapist is *experiencing unconditional positive regard* toward the client.
 5. That the therapist is *experiencing* an *empathic* understanding of the client's *internal frame of reference*.
 6. That the client *perceives*, at least to a minimum degree, conditions 4 and 5, the *unconditional positive regard* of the therapist for him, and the *empathic* understanding of the therapist' (Rogers, 1959, p. 213, original italics).

The fact that Rogers takes the trouble to specify clearly six conditions reflects his desire to define operational criteria that could be tested according to the demands of the positivist scientific research of that time (Mearns and Cooper, 2005). Indeed, much research was conducted in the 1950s and 60s. However, Wilkins (2003) points out that most research was on conditions 3, 4 and 5, often referred to as the 'core conditions' (although this is not Rogers' description). The other conditions have been relatively neglected in terms of research and furthering understanding. Several authors stress the importance of regarding all six con-ditions as a whole, not to be artificially separated. Embleton-Tudor *et al* state that to focus only on the three conditions of congruence, unconditional positive regard and empathy 'compromises the theoretical integrity of the approach as Rogers developed it and left it; it leads to a skewed and partial view of the person-centred approach; and it hinders coherent thinking about and development of person-centred practice' (2004, p. 39). Yet in the nursing literature for example, it is common to see the three core conditions singled out as the main ingredients for therapeutic effectiveness.

The next chapter looks in detail at the conditions of congruence (3), unconditional positive regard (4) and empathy (5), which means I shall say little further about them now. Chapter 9 addresses the condition of establishing contact (1). I will therefore add here a few comments about conditions 2 and 6.

Condition 2 ('that the first person, whom we shall term the client, is in a state of *incongruence*, being *vulnerable* or *anxious*' (Rogers, 1959, p. 213)) is pos-sibly a statement of the obvious but needs to be made explicit. Constructive personality change can only occur as long as there is something that is experienced as not right in the client or threatening to the sense of self, and recognised by the client, however vaguely sensed or poorly articulated. In person-centred terms this is described as a state of incongruence or anxiety, a discrepancy between the experience of the person, or to use Rogers' term, the 'organism', and their self-concept. Anxiety in Rogers' terms may be thought of as meaning psychological disturbance. Embleton-Tudor *et al* suggest that this condition is related to a client's degree of motivation to engage in a process that may bring about change. The greater the awareness (or insight, to use psychiatric terminology) of disturbance, the greater the possibility that a client may want to change. This is in contrast to a client who does not think that anything is amiss. Clearly, such a client is unlikely to engage in or benefit from any formal therapeutic change process.

Condition 6 states that the client must perceive the therapist's unconditional positive regard and empathic understanding to a minimal degree, although Rogers acknowledges the degree as arbitrary. This clearly implies that these conditions are being communicated (to a minimal degree). Perception here is not to be confused with the usual meaning of 'perception' within psychiatry as a term describing the aspect of the mental state relating specifically to the five senses and which, if disturbed, causes illusions or hallucinations. The term perception for Rogers is used synonymously with awareness or consciousness (1959). Thus, the client needs to become aware to some degree of the therapist's unconditional positive regard and empathy, otherwise their communication is in vain. This may require the therapist to check in some way what the client has or has not perceived. I have certainly learnt that it is all too easy to assume that patients are aware of my attitudes and my understanding, only to be shocked that the efforts I went to in communicating them were in vain (although I would actually question whether such communication really is wasted, and certainly *I* often gain in the process of embodying particular attitudes, i.e. it changes me). It is also worth keeping in mind that what is perceived will not simply be the direct product of what is communicated. A host of other influences may come into play such as a person's particular mental state, the context (or environment), or medication. How often, for example, do we consider whether a person is hard of hearing and the impact of this on accurate perception?

Within psychiatric settings I find it is actually very common to encounter people who find the experience and communication of empathy and unconditional positive regard by another person towards them, very overwhelming and threatening. This might lead the experience of these conditions to be denied (not perceived or recognised) or perceived but distorted in some way. This requires mental health professionals to be secure enough in themselves not to feel that they and their efforts are being rejected and to react negatively or punitively.

What perception really involves, from a psychological and philosophical point of view, is an interesting and important question, along with how and why it may become disturbed. What and how are personality factors relevant and how do various psychological disturbances influence perception? For mental health professionals and person-centred therapists then, this condition is worthy of much more attention. It is further explored in Wyatt and Sanders (2002), who see this condition as one about which understanding is very much in development.

The necessary and sufficient conditions for constructive personality change

As well as presenting these conditions in his major 1959 exposition of client-centred therapy, Rogers also presents them, with very slight differences, in a 1957 paper entitled 'The Necessary and Sufficient Conditions of Therapeutic Personality Change'. In this paper he is making a statement about the conditions he regards as effective in all therapies. In other words, the conditions constitute what could be termed an 'integrative framework'. His hypothesis, as the title suggests, is that all six conditions are both 'necessary and sufficient'. I would like to make a few comments about the meaning of this.

In the person-centred community, the issue of whether the conditions are sufficient is one that has been, and continues to be, a source of debate. It is certainly true that therapists practising from other orientations dismiss the notion of the sufficiency of these conditions. A common view is along the lines of Rogers' conditions being a pre-condition for therapy which then involves the application of other skills, specific methods or the 'real work' – a view that irritates many person-centred therapists, particularly when delivered in a patronising way. This issue relates to techniques and interventions, as previously discussed, and the belief that the relationship is subordinate to 'real' professional activities (Borg and Kristiansen, 2004). Suffice it to say though, that if it is believed that techniques or further methods are necessary, then the six conditions alone are thought to be insufficient.

However, I think this issue deserves further reflection. I have certainly been exercised by the meaning of sufficiency within mental health settings and outside the therapy context. As a simple and logical statement I struggle with the notion of sufficiency. The questions I find myself asking are, sufficient for what? What is the goal? Yes, I believe that the conditions are often sufficient for constructive personality change, but is this goal sufficient? In mental health services, personality change alone, as a simply stated goal, is rarely acceptable because of the increasing emphasis on measurable goals and outcomes, on cure of symptoms and solving of problems. Even if such conditions were acknowledged by many mental health professionals as important (let alone 'necessary and sufficient'), it is likely that, as mental health services currently function, they would very rarely be provided in clinical practice. After all, it would also mean abandoning many procedures, techniques and expert interventions and paying attention to the potential healing relationship embodied by the attitudinal conditions already mentioned. It is hard to imagine this being accepted. Bozarth (1998) points out that the fact that so much research looks for specific treatments for specific conditions implies a view that rejects the sufficiency hypothesis. Underlying this is a lack of trust in the capacity and tendency of the person to actualise and to move in the direction of growth and change given certain specified conditions.

To regard the conditions as necessary and sufficient also excludes the possibility of growth occurring outside of a relationship. For Tudor and Worrall it is a 'staggering hypothesis' because it 'rules out the possibility of anyone growing or developing or changing through reading a book, or watching a sunset, or hearing a piece of music, or learning to juggle, or watching a film' (2006, pp. 19–20).

I think where my own trust falters often is not so much in the actualising tendency, but in the capacity of the environment and mental health professionals, including myself, to offer the conditions. My lack of trust is not so much about the potential within patients but about the conditions of mental health settings, which often couldn't be further from being congruent and providing unconditional positive regard and empathic understanding. Simply, the context may not be sufficient for disturbed individuals in need of security, safety and a therapeutic environment in which Rogers' six conditions can be offered.

Tudor and Worrall (2006) also point out that accepting this hypothesis as a logical 'if-then' kind (i.e. change will only happen if these conditions are provided), places disproportionate responsibility for therapy effectiveness and client change on the therapist. It flies in the face of the extra-therapeutic variables (the internal and external resources of the client) that account for 40% of therapeutic effectiveness (Lambert, 1992) as mentioned in Chapter 6.

Despite much research, Rogers' hypothesis of the necessity and sufficiency of all six conditions is not proven, although Wilkins (2003) reminds us that it has not actually been rigorously tested. Nevertheless, the importance of relationship is widely acknowledged. In the person-centred approach the relationship is the therapy and not simply a precursor to therapy.

Conclusion

'We all need to ask ourselves, what kind of a person, showing what kind of commitment, would we want to be "there" for us, were the ship of our lives to founder on the rocks?'

Buchanan-Barker, 2004, p. 10

I know I would want someone who attached primary value to the importance of relationship in their work. It would be someone who had a high level of commitment to seeking to establish connections with patients, who valued the language of 'encounter' with human beings, rather than appointments with patients. This helper would reject the 'therapeutic norm of *under-involvement*' (Thorne, 2002, p. 21, original italics) that short-term approaches and fear of litigation promote. He or she would be prepared to risk criticism from colleagues for being regarded as over-involved and not keeping a 'professional distance', although safeguards such as good supervision and disciplined self-reflection are necessary to be aware of one's own motives and needs.

Unfortunately, in my experience, such mental health professionals are becoming rarer. Working within NHS mental health services, like other institutions, is to risk being contaminated by a culture infected with the 'politics of appearance' (Mearns and Thorne, 2000, p. 41). Not only does it recognise less the value of therapeutic relationships, but the culture undermines the ability of mental health professionals to offer them given the current obsession with measurable activities, cost-effectiveness and short-term working. Managers and politicians seem to me unable to comprehend how vital adequate support and supervision are for all mental health professionals. The result is a workforce who are tired, demoralised and angry and who are unable to offer themselves acceptance and empathy, let alone their patients. I am pessimistic that the current political and cultural climate will recognise the folly of its policies and attitudes before much more human tragedy occurs. In the longer-term I am more optimistic and share the following vision of Mearns and Cooper:

'Whether the change happens by revolution or by evolution, it is inevitable, because it is an essentially untenable position for human beings to seek to deny the centrality of human relationships in their dealings with each other' (2005, p. 164).

However, I am not sure whether this will be in my lifetime and I certainly don't imagine it will happen whilst I am still working in the NHS.

References

Barker P (2000) Reflections on caring as a virtue ethic within an evidence-based culture. *International Journal of Nursing Studies*, **37**: 329–336.

Barrett-Lennard G (2005) *Relationship at the Centre. Healing in a Troubled World.* Whurr Publishers, London.

Bordin E (1994) Theory and research on the therapeutic working alliance: new directions. In A Hovarth and L Greenberg (eds) *The Working Alliance: Theory, Research and Practice.* Wiley, New York.

Borg M and Kristiansen K (2004) Recovery-orientated professionals: Helping relationships in mental health services. *Journal of Mental Health*, **13(5)**: 493–505.

Bozarth J (1998) *Person-Centred Therapy: A Revolutionary Paradigm.* PCCS Books, Ross-on-Wye.

British Medical Association (2003) *Communication skills education for doctors: a discussion paper.* British Medical Association, London.

Buchanan-Barker P (2004) The Tidal Model: uncommon sense. *Mental Health Nursing*, **24(3)**: 6–10.

Clarkson P (2003) *The Therapeutic Relationship* (2nd edition). Whurr Publishers, London.

Department of Health (2004) *The NHS Knowledge and Skills Framework (NHS KSF) and the Development Review Process.* Department of Health, London.

Egan G (2004) *The Skilled Helper: a problem management and opportunity-development approach to helping* (7th edition). Brooks/Cole, Pacific Grove, California.

Embleton-Tudor L, Keemar K, Tudor K, Valentine J and Worrall M (2004) *The Person-Centred Approach. A Contemporary Introduction.* Palgrave Macmillan, Basingstoke.

Freud S (1953) *Civilization, Society and Religion.* The Pelican Freud Library Volume XII. James Strachey (ed). The Hogarth Press, London.

Gask L (2004) *A Short Introduction to Psychiatry.* Sage, London.

Gask L and Usherwood T (2002) The consultation. *British Medical Journal*, **324**: 1567–1569.

Gendlin E (1978) *Focusing.* Bantum Books, New York.

Hirschhorn L (1997) *Reworking Authority. Leading and Following in the Post-Modern Organization.* The MIT Press, Cambridge, MA.

Hovarth A and Bedi R (2002) The alliance. In J Norcross (ed) *Psychotherapy Relationships that Work: Therapist Contributions and Responsiveness to Patients.* Oxford University Press, Oxford, pp. 37–69.

Lambert M (1992) Implications of outcome research for psychotherapy integration. In J Norcross and M Goldfield (eds) *Handbook of Psychotherapy Integration.* Basic Books, New York, pp. 94–129.

Maguire P and Pitceathly C (2002) Key communication skills and how to acquire them. *British Medical Association*, **325**: 697–700.

Mearns D and Thorne B (2000) *Person-Centred Therapy Today. New Frontiers in Theory and Practice.* Sage, London.

Mearns D and Cooper M (2005) *Working at Relational Depth in Counselling and Psychotherapy.* Sage, London.

Natiello P (2001) *The Person-Centred Approach: A passionate presence.* PCCS Books, Ross-on-Wye.

Peck E and Norman I (1999) Working together in adult community mental health services: Exploring inter-professional role relations. *Journal of Mental Health,* **8(3)**: 231–242.

Perlman HH (1979) *Relationship. The Heart of Helping People.* The University of Chicago Press, Chicago.

Reynolds B (2003) Developing therapeutic one-to-one relationships. In P Barker (ed) *Psychiatric and Mental Health Nursing. The craft of caring.* Arnold, London, pp. 139–146.

Rogers C (1957) The Necessary and Sufficient Conditions of Therapeutic Personality Change. *Journal of Consulting Psychology,* **21(2)**: 95–103.

Rogers C (1959) A theory of therapy, personality, and interpersonal relationships, as developed in the client-centred framework. In S Koch (ed) *Psychology: a study of a science. Study 1. Volume 3. Formulations of the person and the social context.* McGraw-Hill, New York, pp. 184–256.

Rogers C (1980) *A Way of Being.* Houghton Mifflin, Boston, MA.

Rogers C (1990) Client-Centred Therapy. In H Kirschenbaum and V Henderson (eds) *Carl Rogers Dialogues.* Constable, London, p. 938. (Original work published 1959)

Roy D (2004) The good psychiatrist. *Psychiatry,* **3(3)**: 5–7.

Sanders P and Wyatt G (2002) The History of Conditions One and Six. In G Wyatt and P Sanders (eds) *Rogers' Therapeutic Conditions: Evolution, Theory and Practice. Volume 4. Contact and Perception.* PCCS Books, Ross-on-Wye, pp. 1–24.

Silverman J, Kurtz S and Draper J (2005) *Skills for Communicating with Patients* (2nd edition). Radcliffe Publishing, Oxford.

Sladden J (2005) Psychotherapy skills in the real world. *British Medical Journal: Career Focus,* **330(7484)**: 33–35.

Stickley T and Freshwater D (2002) The art of loving and the therapeutic relationship. *Nursing Inquiry,* **9(4)**: 250–256.

The Sainsbury Centre for Mental Health (2001) *The Capable Practitioner. A framework and list of the practitioner capabilities required to implement The National Service Framework for Mental Health.* The Sainsbury Centre for Mental Health, London.

Thorne B (2002) *The Mystical Power of Person-Centred Therapy. Hope beyond Despair.* Whurr Publishers, London.

Thorne B (2003) *Carl Rogers* (2nd edition). Sage, London.

Tudor K (1999) 'I'm OK, You're OK – and They're OK': Therapeutic Relationships in Transactional Analysis. In C Feltham (ed) *Understanding the Counselling Relationship.* Sage, London, pp. 90–119.

Tudor K and Worrall M (2006) *Person-Centred Therapy. A Clinical Philosophy.* Routledge, London.

Watkins P (2001) *Mental Health Nursing. The Art of Compassionate Care.* Butterworth-Heinemann, Edinburgh.

Wilkins P (2003) *Person-Centred Therapy in Focus.* Sage, London.

Wyatt G and Sanders P (eds) (2002) *Rogers' Therapeutic Conditions: Evolution, Theory and Practice. Volume 4. Contact and Perception.* PCCS Books, Ross-on-Wye.

Chapter 8

Listening with attitude

'Listening, of this very special, active kind, is one of the most potent forces for change that I know.'

(Rogers, 1990/1986, p. 136)

Introduction

How many times, I wonder, when we are listening to someone are we really just waiting for them to finish speaking so we can then speak? And do we call this listening?

The kind of listening this chapter describes is listening with the *intention* to listen, as a disciplined and active process that can take place within the briefest of conversations or within an hour of therapy. However, this chapter does not include a detailed description of listening skills or techniques. Rather, I shall be discussing the conditions of congruence, unconditional positive regard and empathy (conditions 3, 4 and 5 of Rogers' conditions for constructive personality change, introduced in Chapter 7). Whilst often presented and taught simply as listening skills, they are, if properly understood as Rogers describes them, more accurately regarded as attitudes. And those of us lucky enough to have received them from another, can testify to their transforming potential.

My challenge here is to discuss the above conditions in the context of mental health settings and not just the therapy context, which is the usual context in which they are considered. Therefore, as well as describing each condition from a person-centred point of view, I shall consider the difficulties of putting them into practice within mental health settings, drawing in particular upon my own experiences and challenges. In so doing it should be evident that I regularly experience a large gulf between the ideal and the realities of practising and embodying congruence, unconditional positive regard and empathy. I intend to take each condition in turn, and in the order that Rogers presents them. However, before doing this there are a few further comments I wish to make.

Whilst usually described and considered separately (and indeed Rogers separates them for the purposes of research), these conditions should be conceived of as inter-related. The presence of one depends on the other two. For example, it will be difficult to understand someone empathically without the attitude of unconditional positive regard. If I value someone, it stands to reason that I would want to understand their experience as accurately as possible. In addition, such regard and valuing need to be congruent (i.e. genuine) to be effective and meaningful.

Of Rogers' six conditions, it is these three that usually receive the most attention and are often described as the 'core conditions'. Tudor and Worrall (2006) point out that the term 'core conditions' is misleading, two reasons being that it implies that they are more important than the other three, and that only *they* are necessary and sufficient. Clearly, these conditions could be communicated to a very high degree, but if poorly perceived (condition 6) then their potency will be diminished. This is a reminder of the importance of client factors, which, along with the 'extra-therapeutic variables' (*see* Chapter 6) and the context of the relationship, have a significant influence on how the conditions are perceived and experienced.

Writing about the core conditions, Mearns and Thorne express their irritation with the 'hi-jacking of the concepts into the mainstream of therapeutic practice, without, it would appear, any real understanding of their implications' (2000, p. 85). They are critical of how the conditions are viewed, i.e. as a precursor for the '*real* business of the therapeutic enterprise' indicating, they believe, 'a failure to understand the conditions as the attitudinal expression of a belief system about human nature and development, and about the healing qualities of relation-ship' (p. 85). Undoubtedly, the conditions could be practised as techniques in a superficial way, as is commonly the case within mental health settings, or they could, as Mearns and Thorne say above, be a manifestation of deeply held beliefs about human beings and what we need for growth and healing. Rather than being behavioural strategies to be 'applied', they become a 'way of being', to use Rogers' phrase.

Another implication of the conditions rarely being understood as attitudes is the lack of attention to the importance of self-awareness. Listening that incorporates these attitudes has major implications for personal development. Their quality depends upon the 'person' of the listener and such things as his or her capacity for self-acceptance and empathic sensitivity, qualities which can be developed.

Finally, although I refer to these conditions as attitudes, strictly speaking, unconditional positive regard is most obviously an attitude, whilst congruence describes an 'internal state' and empathy could be regarded as a 'process'. However, collectively they are fundamentally based on attitudes and values towards human beings, the helping process and the importance of relationship and relating.

Congruence

'We must allow ourselves to be moved by others. Psychiatry has lost touch with the ability, indeed it is questionable whether it ever possessed it in the first place. ... We must allow ourselves to be ourselves with others' (Thomas, 1997, p. 242).

What is congruence?

The above statement by Thomas for me captures the essence of congruence. He urges us to be open to our feelings and to be real with others, rather than constructing a façade or behaving in a stereotyped way. Congruence is the state of being oneself in the relationship. It is a way of being that values genuineness and authenticity. Another word sometimes used to describe congruence is trans-parency. Rogers described this as follows:

'In my relationships with persons I have found that it does not help, in the long run, to act as though I were something that I am not' (Rogers, 1995/ 1956, p. 9).

and

'I have not found it to be helpful or effective in my relationships with other people to try to maintain a façade; to act in one way on the surface when I am experiencing something quite different underneath' (*ibid*).

What these various terms for congruence tell us is that this condition includes what we show of ourselves to others – what we communicate verbally and non-verbally. However, congruence is not equivalent to the automatic and spontaneous expression of thoughts and feelings and to self-disclosure. This is a common misunderstanding of congruence. I shall return shortly to the communicative aspect of congruence and to the issue of self-disclosure.

Common misunderstandings of congruence are further fuelled by not appreciating that it fundamentally represents a state within oneself, where a person's 'actual experience [is] accurately represented by his awareness of himself' (Rogers, 1957, p. 97), or where there is 'congruence of self and experience' (Rogers, 1959, p. 206). This way of describing congruence emphasises what McMillan (2004) terms 'intrapersonal congruence', which I describe in Chapter 2. To recap, intrapersonal congruence and incongruence refer to the matching or not between an individual's actual experience and their awareness. The closer the matching, or in Rogers' terms the more accurate the symbolisation in awareness, the more congruent the individual. Put another way, congruence is an awareness of the feelings and the experiences of the organism as they really are, without defensive denial or distortion. This conceptualisation of congruence concerns an inner experience and process. The less defensive I am, the more I am open to the experiences and feelings that flow within me. However, knowing what is going on within me and allowing myself to have my experience as it is depends upon my attitudes towards myself, principally my degree of self-acceptance and ability not to judge negatively my feelings and experiences. Thus it becomes clear how congruence and unconditional positive self-regard are related, a theme to which I shall return in the section on unconditional positive regard.

Putting all the aspects of this multifaceted concept together leads to the following description of congruence by Rogers, albeit in the context of therapy:

'The therapist is openly being the feelings and attitudes that are flowing within at the moment. There is a close matching, or congruence, between what is being experienced at the gut level, what is present in awareness, and what is expressed to the client' (1990/1986, p. 135).

From this description of congruence it is worth pointing out that, certainly within therapy, Rogers is particularly interested in congruence within the relationship. In other words, 'it is not to be expected that the therapist is a completely congruent person at all times' (Rogers, 1959, p. 215).

It is rather unfortunate that such an important concept and key aspect of the person-centred approach can be the cause of confusion. Certainly I have wrestled with it myself. The number of different words Rogers uses to describe it partly contributes to this (Haugh, 2001). In addition, different authors emphasise different facets of congruence, with some focusing on congruence as primarily an internal state and others predominantly focusing on how congruence is expressed. This illustrates what Lietaer identifies as the 'two sides: an inner and an outer one' (2001a, p. 36). Possibly it is difficult for mental health professionals to view it as an internal state (albeit one that has behavioural consequences), preferring simply to see congruence as a communication skill or form of behaviour.

Congruence in practice

One of the commitments and challenges for me in seeking to become more congruent is the development of certain attitudes towards myself that will then enable me to acknowledge and experience difficult feelings and thoughts towards myself, others and the world. If I have a sufficiently high degree of self-acceptance and I am warmly disposed towards myself as a person, then it is more likely that I will be able to allow into my awareness painful and difficult emotions such as fear, anxiety, sadness, despair and confusion. Tudor and Worrall describe one of the requirements of congruence as being able 'to acknowledge and accept our own fears, failings and vulnerabilities, and to risk feeling or being incongruent and disintegrated' (2006, p. 233).

Of course, emotional reactions may not be directed towards anyone, but what about negative reactions towards other people such as boredom, irritation, jealousy, anger or contempt? Furthermore, if I hold a strong belief that all human beings are basically of value, how do I manage strong feelings of revulsion or hostility to the degree that I might even feel destructive towards that individual and want to inflict harm in some way?

These questions lead to a discussion of 'interpersonal congruence', or outer congruence, to use McMillan's and Lietaer's distinctions respectively. This is the aspect of congruence concerned with what we communicate to others. It includes the tricky issue of self-disclosure of thoughts, feelings and perceptions, which can cause considerable dilemmas for person-centred practitioners, and indeed anyone who is interested in being genuine and transparent. Rogers (1957) considers the degree of what to communicate of himself to the client a 'puzzling matter', although I think the key word here may be 'degree' rather than 'what'.

As previously stated, being congruent is not the same as self-disclosure, but what we may or may not self-disclose does relate to congruence. What is most essential to consider in any discussion of self-disclosure is the context. For example, what I choose to disclose will depend on the nature of the relationship and whether I am relating to friends, colleagues, patients, clients, acquaintances or strangers. Furthermore, within a helping role it will be important to consider the potential impact of what I disclose of my thoughts and feelings on the particular patient or client at that particular time. I have wondered what my colleagues, patients and clients, both past and present, would make of my self-disclosures in this book and whether they will be experienced as helpful or unhelpful (although if I am honest I have considered more the potential consequences, both positive and negative, for me as a person and professional in what I have chosen to self-disclose). This then, is one of the questions that I ask myself when considering what and when to self-disclose: for whose benefit and if it is for mine, partly or solely, is this acceptable? It is important to consider in what way self-disclosures may be interpreted, bearing in mind that often it is a case of best guessing and taking a considered risk or not. For example, one person might treat my self-disclosure as a measure of my trust and respect for that person, whilst another might regard it as an unwanted invasion into their space and a distraction from their agenda. I am generally much more disciplined about what I choose to reveal of my thoughts and feelings within work contexts compared to other settings.

Some of the most difficult dilemmas, particularly when in a helping role, concern when to communicate what we commonly consider to be negative feelings, especially feelings towards our patients such as anger, irritation, impatience and frustration. Writing in the context of a therapy relationship, Mearns and Thorne offer some guidance here. For them, as for Rogers, when experiencing feelings relevant to the client 'which are *persistent* or particularly *striking*' (1999, p. 92, original italics) it may well be appropriate to voice them. For example, if I am aware of a regular feeling of irritation when a client talks about a particular subject, such that I find I cannot concentrate on what he or she is saying because I am preoccupied with my feeling of irritation, it is probably necessary that I voice my feeling. However, I need to pay careful attention to the way I do so. Telling my client I find him or her irritating would clearly not be helpful, as well as inaccurate. Far more constructive and accurate would be to say something along the lines of my noticing feelings within myself when he or she is talking about a certain subject (owning my feeling and taking responsibility for it), and perhaps saying either that I am curious about it, or that I feel I should voice it because I am aware that I struggle to listen as well as I would like to. In other words, disclosing my feeling of irritation springs from a concern that this feeling is affecting my listening. It demonstrates a desire to take care of the relationship. Clearly what this calls for then, is an awareness of what feelings and thoughts I am experiencing when with another so that I can spot when they may be interfering with empathy and unconditional positive regard. Such self-awareness allows me to spot various biases and prejudices that might render my expression of warmth and acceptance less real and genuine. How this translates to non-therapy relationships, and to the day-to-day practice of mental health professionals, is the topic for the next section.

Congruence in mental health settings

I wonder what I would be like if I were congruent at all times when in the work place. Whilst congruence is my aspiration, I acknowledge that I am often far from being in touch with my feelings and inner experiences (positive and negative) as they arise throughout the course of the day. Certainly there is often a discrepancy between what I communicate to others of my thoughts and feelings and what I am actually thinking and feeling. I suggest that this is actually the norm for most mental health professionals. This is where it is important to acknowledge just what an awesome challenge it is to be congruent within mental health settings, both when with our patients and with colleagues, or whilst conducting the other myriad tasks expected of us. I think working in mental health settings, as they are currently structured and resourced, places particularly heavy demands where congruence is concerned. It is an environment, as highlighted in previous chapters, that can create intolerable pressures, frustrations and tensions. In the current climate of rapid and sweeping changes to the way services are organised, working in an environment of widespread demoralisation, confusion and other difficult emotions is potentially so overwhelming that in order to function effectively it seems necessary to keep many negative feelings out of conscious awareness much of the time. Yet, defending against powerful and negative emotions, certainly in the long run, is likely to be harmful for mental health professionals, as well as patients on the receiving end of such incongruence.

What though, might the consequences be of showing our vulnerabilities, being open about our fears, uncertainties and weaknesses? Within the medical profession a culture of stoicism and fear of admitting vulnerability is clearly apparent. It becomes easy to hide behind the professional masks we learn to wear, often in the name of emotional detachment that is taught as the mark of a good professional. Yet, if mental health professionals are not able to be congruent, what right have we to expect and hope that our patients develop greater congruence? It is a tragic irony that the incongruence of mental disturbance is often met by the incongruence of mental health professionals, perpetuating the very disturbance in patients that we are trying to treat.

I also recognise incongruence in my own work by virtue of not fully practising from my own values and belief systems about what is most important in mental health care. I find myself following procedures and processes that I do not believe in philosophically and ethically. This sets up considerable tensions and frustrations that have major implications for how I am and what I communicate within the workplace.

Finally in this section I want to consider particular challenges to being congruent when with patients, especially the issue of self-disclosure. How do I behave when I experience hostile feelings, or exasperation, or strong dislike towards patients? Is it right that I keep such feelings to myself, or perhaps only share them with colleagues? I think this is where making some assessment of the degree of intensity of such feelings is important, as well as assessing the potential impact of these feelings on patients even if expressed only non-verbally because it is impossible to hide them. This is where supervision becomes important to explore the origin of negative reactions towards patients and to become more aware of how our own life experiences give rise to prejudices and judgemental attitudes. It may also be important to consider limiting our responsibilities and interactions with those patients who evoke strongly negative emotional reactions in us that cannot be worked through in supervision, calling on colleagues to share or take over responsibility. Unfortunately, such actions may be interpreted as a failure to cope, rather than as a mature response to emotional realities that may damage patients if ignored. The fear of being perceived as failing is probably one of the reasons we choose to ignore or deny our difficulties with some patients.

Within a therapy context, however, or when I do not have the option of sharing or handing over my role to others, how do I manage difficult feelings and do I disclose them? The answer is that probably I would have to find a way of voicing them, obviously taking care of how I do so and out of concern for the quality of the relationship. However, for those mental health professionals whose contacts with patients are brief and when there is not a heavy investment in the relationship, it may not be appropriate or necessary to disclose difficult and uncomfortable reactions. Exploring them in supervision would still be useful though.

There is one particular instance when I am often caught in the dilemma of how to respond to patients. This concerns the issue of hope and its opposite: despair. What do I communicate when I do not feel hopeful about someone's future? It is important to state here that my lack of hope is usually more to do with my feelings and beliefs about the mental health service and society in general than my beliefs about a person's innate healing and recovery potential. This issue is particularly significant when one of the core attributes for psychiatrists is bringing 'encouragement and hope to patients and their carers' (Royal College of Psychiatrists, 2000, p. 5), and mental health professionals who convey hope are often valued by patients (Borg and Kristiansen, 2004). Yet if I don't feel hopeful how can I instil hope without being incongruent? This issue is worthy of more exploration than space here allows, particularly concerning the nature of hope. Is it an emotion, a belief, a cognitive process, a statement of faith, or a mixture? Suffice it to say though, that I believe congruence is still important. I also need to be as clear as possible about what might be contributing to my feelings of hopelessness, such as my general mood and whether other factors not relevant to the patient are intruding.

The value of congruence

'Mystery evokes the illusion of power, transparency dissolves it.' (Mearns and Thorne, 1999, p. 97)

Given what I have discussed in this book about power, it stands to reason that one of the values of congruence for person-centred practitioners is its capacity to reduce the power imbalance in the helping relationship. Related to this is the increased likelihood of gaining a patient's trust when I am able to demystify psychiatry and my role as a mental health professional by being as genuine as possible. The more I can avoid erecting a professional façade, the more likely it is that I will be trusted. Likewise, the more I am honest and straight with people, for example, acknowledging my uncertainties and not being afraid to say 'I don't know', the more likely it is that I will be trusted. Falseness, professional masks, devotion to being the role rather than being a person with a role, can make one less likely to be trusted.

Being genuine is also the basis of unconditional positive regard and empathy, as well as being an expression of valuing the other person. Taking risks for the sake of the relationship (congruence can at times feel highly risky) demonstrates a valuing of that relationship.

Finally, referring to therapy, Spinelli (2005) notes that a congruent therapist can also act as a role model for authenticity. Congruence in the therapist encourages congruence in clients. I think this could equally apply to mental health professionals and their patients and colleagues.

Unconditional positive regard

'Inviting and allowing another person to have his or her experience just as it is – this is perhaps the greatest gift anyone can offer.' (Welwood, 2000, p. 144)

Understanding unconditional positive regard

Lietaer (2001b) points out that unconditional positive regard is a multidimensional concept. Like congruence then, it is not a concept that is simple and easy to grasp and different authors offer different perspectives. Also like congruence, Rogers uses a number of words to describe it, one of the most common being 'acceptance'. Other words and expressions he uses include 'prizing', 'non-possessive caring', 'warmth', 'respect' and 'confirmation' of persons (confirmation being a word and idea he borrowed from the theologian Martin Buber). Still other words are used by contemporary authors and person-centred practitioners. Mearns and Cooper use the word 'affirmation' quite deliberately to emphasise an active process of prizing, indicating that 'it is far more than simply refraining from judgement, or holding an attitude of "however you are is alright by me". Here, there is a positive affirmation of the client down to the very essence of their being, a confirmation of their uniqueness, individuality and humanity' and 'a deep valuing of how they are in the world' (2005, p. 43).

Already it is possible to see how different words can convey subtle or not so subtle nuances of meaning and emphasis. Affirming the value of persons and conveying warmth, to me, feel different from simple respect and acceptance. Acceptance, to me, also feels close to tolerance or resignation. However, the following descriptive passages by Rogers of unconditional positive regard leave little doubt about what he means by this attitude. It:

> 'involves the therapist's willingness for the client to be whatever immediate feeling is going on – confusion, resentment, fear, anger, courage, love, or pride. It is nonpossessive caring' (1990/1986, p. 136);

and

> 'as much feeling of acceptance for the client's expression of negative, "bad", painful, fearful, defensive, abnormal feelings as for his expression of "good", positive, mature, confident, social feelings, as much acceptance of ways in which he is inconsistent as of ways in which he is consistent. It means a caring for the client, but not in a possessive way or in such a way as simply to satisfy the therapist's own needs. It means a caring for the client as a *separate* person, with permission to have his own feelings, his own experiences' [original italics] (1990/1957, p. 225).

Two aspects which these descriptions highlight are first, how unconditional positive regard is a caring and positive response, and second, the unconditional nature of positive regard. Like Mearns and Cooper's use of the word 'affirming', Rogers emphasises how this attitude is far from neutral. It is not simply respect without any emotional involvement. It is not just the absence of negative judgements. It is also more than having a positive feeling about someone and it cannot simply be equated with affection and liking. Unconditional positive regard goes much deeper than an emotional experience towards a person. It is part of one's value system and belief that human beings are worthy of valuing, regardless of their behaviours. In other words, this attitude does not waver and cannot simply be turned on and off. Lietaer describes unconditionality as meaning 'that I keep on *valuing the deeper core of the person, what she potentially is and can become'* (2001b, pp. 92–93, original italics). Needless to say though, experiencing positive regard unconditionally can be difficult and often impossible to attain. I shall discuss such difficulties and challenges shortly.

I would like to make a few more comments before next turning to why this attitude is important. Rogers suggests that unconditional positive regard is a rather unfortunate phrase because it implies an 'all-or-nothing' quality. Like most of the other conditions, this one also occurs in degrees. It is also important that it is *perceived* by the client or patient in order to be effective, although this does not necessarily depend upon particular communication skills. It is enough that this attitude is experienced by the helper or listener and it will be conveyed by its very existence. However, it is often empathic understanding that acts as the vehicle by which this attitude is communicated. Put another way, it is empathic understanding that expresses it, or as Rogers puts it, unconditional positive regard 'does not mean much until it involves understanding' (1967, p. 34). It is important to bear in mind that I cannot really know someone whilst I am judging them. This illustrates the connectedness of unconditional positive regard and empathy.

The importance of unconditional positive regard

'The curious paradox is that when I accept myself as I am, then I change ... we cannot change, we cannot move away from what we are, until we thoroughly *accept* what we are. Then change seems to come about unnoticed.' (Rogers, 1995/1956, p. 10)

This observation by Rogers asserts that unconditional positive regard is the key to change. Bozarth describes it as the 'primary change agent' (1998, p. 47). What change then, does it facilitate? Put simply, unconditional positive regard dissolves the 'conditions of worth' that keep a person from being in touch with their actual experience and from being congruent. A detailed description of conditions of worth and the development of incongruence is found in Chapter 2. To recap briefly, it is theorised that human beings' powerful need for positive regard sets up conditions of worth, whereby we experience and allow into our awareness only those emotions, thoughts and perceptions that are most likely to bring positive regard from others, or to avoid negative regard. Thus, we select the experiences we allow into our awareness according to those conditions of worth. In so doing we become cut off from our actual experiences and our defences ensure that we are and remain incongruent.

A common condition of worth is that feeling low in mood or expressing sadness is not acceptable. Perhaps this is a result of what parents communicate to their children when growing up, and is reinforced by cultural attitudes that encourage us to remember that there are always people worse off, that we should be content with our lot and that anything less is unacceptable self-pity. In order, then, to avoid negative judgements, a person may learn to 'bury' or dismiss feelings of sadness or despondency when they arise (*see* Rogers' defence mechanisms of denial and distortion, also in Chapter 2) and will want to avoid such feelings and certainly avoid communicating them. However, by perceiving unconditional positive regard from another, a person may come to believe that he or she will still be accepted whatever he or she feels. Previous defences against feeling sad or despondent will automatically be challenged, allowing exploration and expression of feelings that were previously experienced as shameful or confusing. Unconditional positive regard gives a person freedom to explore feelings, thoughts and perceptions without the fear of negative judgements. It may allow a person to become more deeply in touch with his or her inner experiences and therefore more integrated and congruent. It may also dissolve feelings of worthlessness by endowing a person with a sense of worth.

This attitude is particularly important, essential even, within mental health settings because many patients experience a profound sense of worthlessness. This is especially the case for the high prevalence of patients who have been the victims of childhood abuse – emotional, physical and sexual. Common psychotic experiences include hearing voices of a judgemental and derogatory nature, delusions of persecution or ideas of guilt. Many patients have also been on the receiving end of negative judgements by virtue of having a mental illness or having been in contact with mental health professionals. Stigma remains prevalent within our society. Many people feel a sense of shame or embarrassment concerning their mental experiences and mental health professionals are in a key position to offer acceptance and understanding, perhaps experienced for the first time by some patients. Tragically, in my opinion, unconditional positive regard is in short supply within mental health settings, an issue I shall be considering in the next section.

Unconditional positive regard in mental health settings

Having briefly asserted the value of this attitude, it cannot be overstated, in my opinion, that there are considerable challenges to cultivating it within mental health settings. This section aims to highlight some of these.

The very goals of psychiatric treatment and mental health care could be experienced and perceived as a major condition of worth in which the patient is more acceptable, in their own and others' eyes, without their symptoms and having responded to interventions. The goal of mental health care is to effect change. This will make it difficult for many patients to experience being equally acceptable as persons with or without their symptoms and behaviours. I notice how affirming and encouraging my responses to patients are when they report improvement. Because I feel heartened, I am often more open and accepting in my behaviours towards these patients than towards those who consistently show minimal signs of change. It is not uncommon for patients to tell their psychiatrist or nurse that they are improving in order to avoid disapproval when reporting lack of 'progress'. This expectation of improvement contrasts with Rogers' attitude of acceptance, out of which change may then occur, as the earlier quote by Rogers expresses. Mental health and mental state then, are major conditions of worth, not just within mental health settings but also in society generally.

Given how powerful (and perfectly laudable) a desire it is in most mental health professionals for patients to get better and for mental suffering to be relieved, it becomes natural to focus on the mental experiences of patients such as their symptoms and behaviours. One of the difficulties of cultivating unconditional positive regard for the whole person is that often we are focusing on psychopathology, how to categorise it, and therefore what diagnosis to give the patient. We learn to see aspects of the patient rather than the whole person.

This is a clear example of the influence of the reductionist, scientific culture on mental health professionals.

Another difficulty in developing unconditional positive regard is overcoming the commonly taught guideline that we should judge the behaviour and not the person. In other words, we are taught to separate the person from their behaviour, particularly when those behaviours are unpleasant or destructive to self or others. I agree with Tudor and Worrall who suggest that this is both naïve and an unhelpful 'artificial splitting'. For them 'a person *is* his behaviour' (2006, p. 134), and our task is to understand the environmental influences on such behaviour.

At this point, perhaps it is important that I remind myself that I am probably not capable of achieving complete unconditional positive regard, especially towards people who are hostile or who have committed abominable acts or who generally behave in antisocial ways. Wilkins also helpfully suggests that 'perhaps the first thing each of us needs to accept is that our ability to offer unconditional positive regard is limited; the second is to discover those limits and to seek to expand them (while working within them in the interim)' (2001, p. 46). This is where self-awareness is important, as well as seeking or taking opportunities for personal reflection such as supervision.

It is also important that I remind myself that I can extend unconditional positive regard towards someone without approving of or agreeing with their behaviours. Nevertheless, I am aware of certain behaviours of individuals that leave me experiencing judgemental and negative attitudes towards them, particularly patient behaviours that have consequences for other patients and the service. A good example is when patients manipulate services for their own ends, e.g. cheating the social security system, or who waste resources by not attending appointments (out of lack of respect for services rather than as a consequence of their particular health problems such as poor memory). I also sometimes find it difficult to accept patients who sabotage efforts to help them, even when I might understand why they should do so. Likewise, I think mental health professionals generally struggle to accept patients who adopt the sick role. It seems that a powerful condition of worth is that patients are more acceptable if they *want* to 'get better' and are motivated. Such motivation is judged according to whether patients follow the advice of mental health professionals and willingly accept the treatment interventions offered.

I notice a theme developing here and it revolves around the issue of responsibility. I am often liable to feel negative towards people who cannot or will not take responsibility for how they behave and for their mental well-being, particularly when they attempt to hold me mainly responsible for their well-being. Unfortunately, society and the government are currently placing unreasonable responsibilities on mental health professionals and services, trying to hold us responsible for social ills and ready and eager to blame us when things go wrong. This pressure and sense of responsibility can become so great that they lead to negative judgements towards those patients for whom we are expected, unreasonably, to be heavily responsible.

There are clearly issues here that mental health professionals working for a public service deal with that do not generally concern privately practising person-centred therapists whose services are sought and work contracted, and for which clients pay. I recognise my difficulties in accepting patients who waste the limited resources that the NHS has and whose behaviours, therefore, have direct consequences on other patients. One of the extra pressures with which mental health professionals deal is rationing limited resources and making decisions according to which patients are most likely to use services responsibly and benefit from them. This puts me in the position of making predictions about the likely effects of an intervention and it is something that I regularly feel uncomfortable doing. Not only may I be wrong in my predictions, but it also seems unfair and unreasonable not to give patients the benefit of the doubt.

I notice how much my sense of feeling burdened can quickly lead to feelings of resentment, especially when the burden feels unreasonable or I receive little support with it because colleagues are already carrying their own burdens. Institutional pressures and expectations and lack of support play a large part in contributing to feeling burdened. I regularly recognise how this experience interferes with, and limits, my capacity to develop unconditional positive regard. This is particularly the case towards patients with dependency needs and behaviours, even when I regard dependency as being a legitimate mental health need for many patients. If caring is a dimension of unconditional positive regard then it is threatened when mental health professionals experience what is commonly referred to as 'compassion fatigue'. Environmental factors (i.e. the working environment) are, I believe, some of the biggest obstacles for mental health professionals in developing unconditional positive regard, as well as developing congruence and empathy.

Another formidable obstacle though, is the degree to which we accept ourselves. I wonder how many mental health professionals would rate their self-esteem as generally low for much of the time, including when in the workplace. From my own observations, I would suggest that this is the case for a significant proportion of the mental health workforce, regardless of profession. By self-esteem I also mean self-acceptance. In addition, it is usually the case that we find it difficult to accept in others what we cannot accept in ourselves and we may be unaware of what aspects of ourselves we are struggling to accept. Rogers stresses the importance of self-acceptance, whilst recognising that this is not an easy path:

> '[If] I can form a helping relationship to myself – if I can be sensitively aware of and acceptant towards my own feelings – then the likelihood is great that I can form a helping relationship toward another ... It has meant that if I am to facilitate the personal growth of others in relation to me, then I must grow, and while this is often painful it is also enriching.' (1990/1958, p. 120)

This is where good supervision becomes so important. Not only may we become more aware of our prejudices and how our own histories and experiences influence our attitudes, but we may also have an opportunity to develop greater self-acceptance. However, this depends also upon the attitudes of the supervisor towards the supervisee and whether the supervisor is capable of unconditional positive regard and values it as an important dimension of the supervisory process.

Final comments ...

In advocating the transforming potential of unconditional positive regard, it is important, however, to be aware that for many patients whose personality development has been heavily influenced by conditions of worth and whose self-loathing is profound, the experience of this attitude from mental health professionals may be threatening, frightening or simply incomprehensible. Unconditional positive regard may therefore be rejected initially as a person tries to defend their self-concept that believes they are unworthy of positive regard. For other patients it may take a long time to trust that positive regard is unconditional and isn't something sinister and that it is not going to lead to betrayal or some other manipulation. It is for patients such as these that relationships with mental health professionals need a long time to become established and for whom time-limited interventions are often wholly inappropriate and an example of the superficiality and inadequacy of much mental health practice, including psychological therapy.

In writing about unconditional positive regard as a 'change agent', I am aware that it is in competition with other interventions such as medication. This raises interesting questions concerning the interface between biological and psychological models of understanding our mental processes. Can congruence and self-acceptance be translated into biochemical terms? Given the reliance on medication and psychological techniques within mental health settings, unconditional positive regard is rarely voiced as a credible alternative or addition. I therefore ask myself what can be done to raise the profile of this desperately needed attitude within mental health settings – an attitude that any professional can embody.

Empathy

'The next time you get into an argument with your wife, or your friend, or with a small group of friends, just stop the discussion for a moment and for an experiment, institute this rule. "Each person can speak up for himself only *after* he has first restated the ideas and feelings of the previous speaker accurately, and to that speaker's satisfaction." You see what this would mean. It would simply mean that before presenting your own point of view, it would be necessary for you to really achieve the other speaker's frame of reference – to understand his thoughts and feelings so well that you could summarise them for him. Sounds simple, doesn't it? But if you try it you will discover it is one of the most difficult things you have ever tried to do.' (Rogers, 1967, p. 332)

A person-centred view of empathy

Not only can empathy be difficult to practise, as Rogers suggests with the above challenge, but as a concept it is not as simple to understand as one might be led to believe given how regularly the word is used (without description or definition) in health care settings. In this section I want to explore the concept of empathy, both how it is commonly viewed, and how it is understood from a person-centred perspective.

Ask mental health professionals to define empathy and a frequent response may well be to describe it using the metaphor of 'stepping into a person's shoes'. Other metaphors often used are 'getting into someone's skin' or 'seeing the world through another's eyes'. The fact that metaphors help to describe empathy might seem to indicate that capturing its essence with a more formal use of words or definition is actually very difficult. Dictionary definitions do of course exist, such as 'the power of identifying oneself mentally with (and so fully comprehending) a person or object of contemplation' (Oxford English Reference Dictionary, 1996), but person-centred empathy would not agree with either the notion of 'identifying' with or 'fully comprehending'.

So what is empathy? How do we know if someone is empathising with us? For me it is when I feel I have been understood accurately (not necessarily perfectly or totally) and arriving at such an understanding has been the *intention* of the other person. They have made some effort to enter into my world of feelings, thoughts and meanings. Already identified then, are two facets of empathy: it is a *process* and it involves *understanding.* In this respect the term 'empathic understanding' is probably more suitable. For Worrall, empathic understanding 'embraces the detail of understanding, which is a cognitive process, as well as the warmth of accepting, which is an affective one' (2001, p. 216). He goes on to describe the concept as 'a disciplined process that involves both thinking and feeling, and one that attends to both the thinking and feeling life of the other' (*ibid*). Here are two more aspects of a person-centred perspective on empathy: it is a *disciplined* process (which links up with the intentional aspect of it) and it has both *cognitive and emotional* components.

However accurately I might sense the experiences and perceptions of the other person though, this will not have any impact on them unless this understanding is communicated. One might say then, that empathy involves two ongoing processes – understanding and communicating that understanding. Considerable skill may be involved in the communicative aspects of empathy, particularly to avoid giving the impression that all one is doing is simply 'reflecting feelings' in a mechanical way. Before moving on to explore these communicative aspects and something of the method of empathy, I would like to capture further the person-centred essence of empathy. Rather, I would like to highlight how Rogers describes empathy. The following passage is taken from a chapter in which he re-evaluates empathy, trying to correct frequent misunderstandings that it is little more than a superficial set of techniques. It is aptly titled 'Empathic: An Unappreciated Way of Being' and is one of his most comprehensive descriptions:

'An empathic way of being with another person has several facets. It means entering the private perceptual world of the other and becoming thoroughly at home in it. It involves being sensitive, moment by moment, to the changing felt meanings which flow in this other person, to the fear or rage or tenderness or confusion or whatever that he or she is experiencing. ... It includes communicating your sensings of the person's world as you look with fresh and unfrightened eyes at elements of which he or she is fearful. It means frequently checking with the person as to the accuracy of your sensings, and being guided by the responses you receive. You are a confident companion to the person in his or her inner world. ... To be with another in this way means that for the time being, you lay aside your own views and values in order to enter another's world without prejudice. In some sense it means that you lay aside your self; this can only be done by persons who are secure enough in themselves that they know they will not get lost in what may turn out to be the strange or bizarre world of the other, and that they can comfortably return to their own world when they wish. ... Perhaps this description makes clear that being empathic is a complex, demanding, and strong – yet a subtle and gentle – way of being.' (1980, pp. 142–143)

Here is another often quoted passage in which Rogers describes empathy in the form of questions to himself:

'Can I let myself enter fully into the world of his feelings and personal meanings and see these as he does? Can I step into his private world so completely that I lose all desire to evaluate or judge it? Can I enter it so sensitively that I can move about in it freely, without trampling on meanings which are precious to him? Can I sense it so accurately that I can catch not only the meanings of his experience which are obvious to him, but those meanings which are only implicit, which he sees only dimly or as confusion? Can I extend this understanding without limit?' (1967, p. 53)

For me, these passages, which deserve quoting at length, capture a breath-taking sensitivity and compassion, as well as a total readiness to hear, sense and understand whatever it is a person might be experiencing. He communicates through these descriptions his deep desire to connect with persons, and in such a way that demonstrates a belief in their inestimable worth. Can I, too, embody this 'way of being'?

How to be empathic

Plenty of texts already exist that describe and aim to facilitate deeper understanding and development of the practice of empathy. They vary according to whether they are written specifically to present a person-centred perspective (e.g. Vincent's 'Being Empathic. A companion for counsellors and therapists' (2005)), whether discussing empathy in the context of counselling and psychotherapy (e.g. Vincent again), whether empathy is being presented as an emotional skill useful for doctors (Halpern, 2001), or whether as primarily a communication skill (e.g. Egan's 'The Skilled Helper' (2004)). Clearly then, discussions and descriptions on how to be empathic depend on the audience and how the concept is primarily understood, including its purpose and value. This section aims to give a further flavour of person-centred empathy by focusing on what is involved (empathic method) and on the communication of empathy.

At this point it may be useful to draw attention to the related concept of 'sympathy'. What is happening when we are offering our sympathies to someone? Sympathy has been likened to sending condolences or commiserations. It has also been described as 'the state of being simultaneously affected with a feeling similar or corresponding to that of another; the act of sharing in or responding to an emotion, sensation, or condition of another person' (Oxford English Reference Dictionary, 1996).

Of notice here is its description as a 'state'. This definition of sympathy also implies that it is largely an emotional response. Sympathy also usually involves some degree of compassion and a feeling *for* someone (rather than *with*), or of being touched emotionally by their experience or predicament. However, where it crucially differs from empathy is in how much our responses and feelings are guided by our own experiences when sympathising, in contrast to putting aside our own experience to imagine the situation as the other person might be experiencing it when empathising. Sympathy is represented by the very common response 'I know what you mean'.

An example here may be useful. Grief is a universal experience and it is probably the death of a loved one that is one of the most common reasons for 'sending our sympathies' or communicating sympathy. What often happens though, is that we find ourselves imagining how we might feel if we lost a loved one, or even recalling how we felt having been through the grieving process ourselves. We may feel sadness for the anticipated emptiness or numbness we remember feeling, which we imagine the other person will feel. In other words, even though sympathy involves a connection of feeling (the value of which, incidentally, should not be dismissed), it arises out of imagining and assuming the feelings, thoughts and perceptions of the bereaved person based on how we would feel and experience the same situation.

Whilst it is true that common human experiences such as grief have particular characteristics such that it may be appropriate at times to talk about the commonalities of human experience, nevertheless, each person's experience of grief will be unique. Too often we tend to assume that we know what another's experience is or will be. Empathy, in contrast to sympathy, assumes the uniqueness of a person's experience. It involves imagining how the experience is for that particular person, at that particular time, given their life story, their personality, their circumstances and all the individual and unique meanings that such a grief will hold for that person. Clearly then, it takes a great deal more effort and is a more involved activity than sympathy. As Embleton-Tudor *et al* put it, 'Empathy demands that we attempt to understand not only the meaning, but also the nuances of feeling, the value and the significance which the other person attaches to the subject under discussion' (2004, p. 143), whether this is bereavement or other grief, or even good experiences such as being offered a much wanted job.

I think empathy also involves an essential humility. It is adopting a position of not knowing, whilst also involving a preparedness and desire to understand as accurately as possible the unique and subtle features of a person's experience. Purton provides a good example of how much subtler our experience is than that which general concepts imply. 'For example', he says, 'suppose that a person is in a state which may correctly be described as "angry". That is an application of a general concept. Yet there is more to that person's experience: they *are* angry, but with an undercurrent of hurt, and not even exactly angry, but more full of resentment in connection with what was done to them, yet also angry with *themself* for letting it happen, and upset because they have let this happen *again* when they had only yesterday realised that this is what they always let happen. . . .' (2004, p. 51, original italics).

I shall turn now to the communication of empathy and explore what person-centred empathic skills are, as well as how they are commonly described and understood in non-person-centred literature. The latter often leads to unhelpful caricatures of various techniques. Although it is accurate to talk about the skill of empathy, I notice myself slightly flinching at the use of the word 'skill', for reasons that will become apparent. Given what I have previously discussed concerning empathy involving a position of not knowing, yet imagining what an experience is like for that particular person in their unique situation, it is necessary to be tentative when we think we have understood what a person means. We need to check out our understanding, particularly if we rely on our intuition. Thus, when I respond to someone along the lines of 'I get the idea that for you not being able to help out in the family business at this time is particularly troubling because this is one of the few things you feel you can do to show your family how much you care. ...', I would try to do so in a gentle, questioning manner, checking that I am making the correct assumptions and guessing accurately something of the feeling, although I may still not know what to feel 'troubled' might really be like for that person. Furthermore, if I am responding and checking my understanding in the most helpful way, then I will also be giving the person an opportunity to clarify, elaborate or correct my misunderstanding.

Unfortunately, all too often in my view, empathy is taught as a technique or behavioural response, such as 'reflecting feelings' or using the well-worn phrase 'I hear what you're saying'. Empathy is often referred to as simply a communication skill without reference to attitudes or values. Egan (2004), for example, emphasises the techniques of empathy, describing it as involving, for example, perceptiveness and assertiveness. He suggests helpers learn certain responses in the form of 'You feel ... because ...'. Such phrases may be useful but unfortunately they encourage a stereotyped response system in which the listener relies on a stock of phrases, rather than on genuine empathic sensitivity and understanding that try to sense the other person's experience in all its uniqueness. Incidentally, it is easy to spot stereotyped empathic responses (along with other communication skills) in non-health care settings. They are used, for example, in the world of sales and marketing and taught to employees as 'tricks of the trade' to influence customers. Empathy that is not genuine (i.e. there is no real interest in the other person) and without unconditional positive regard is shallow and unhelpful. Yet this is often the outcome of teaching empathy simply as a communication skill. It also leads to some damaging caricatures of the person-centred therapist who, as Vincent describes, 'has a bouncy rubber spring for a neck, and simply sits there nodding and bobbing sagely, interjecting the occasional (but well-timed) "hm-mm" and "uh-huh"!' (2005, p. 85).

However, to deny that the communication of empathy requires specific skills is equally unhelpful because this implies that it is easy and doesn't require development within the practitioner. It requires a level of attentiveness and concentration that is often difficult to achieve, particularly in environments full of distractions such as hospital wards and badly sound-proofed clinic rooms. It also requires laying aside the desire to explain, evaluate and categorise the patient's experience, a particular challenge for mental health professionals. It is not being interested in understanding *about*, which is the objective stance (*see* Chapter 5), although empathy is taught to psychiatrists 'as a method or a tool' (Sims, 2003, p. 14) in order 'to *measure* another person's internal subjective experience' (Sims, 2003, p. 3, my italics). A person-centred view of empathy is very different from psychiatric descriptions of empathy as a method of (largely intellectual) understanding in order to diagnose. Rather, empathy from the person-centred point of view could be described as a process of understanding *with*.

Nevertheless, it is possible to talk about empathic method or, rather, a method of achieving the openness to experience that is an essential aspect of empathy.

We may draw upon phenomenological thinking in which three 'rules' have been described that allow us to approach subjective experience with openness (*see* Spinelli, 2005). The first is described as *bracketing* our own experience. This involves putting to one side all our biases, prejudices, judgements, evaluations, expectations and assumptions, and is what Rogers means when he describes empathy as a laying aside of one's self (see the earlier quote). The second rule is only to *describe* experience and not analyse or judge it. This will enable meaning to emerge from the experience rather than as something imposed from outside. Finally, we need to resist putting experiences in an order of importance but to treat them all with *equal* value. This means paying as much attention to the seemingly smaller details of a person's behaviour as to the bigger gestures. However, it needs to be acknowledged that we can never follow these rules completely. It seems natural to place experiences in some form of hierarchy and to analyse them, as well as impossible to view experience without it being influenced to some degree by our biases, viewpoints and assumptions. Nevertheless, being aware of these tendencies will help us to approach experience in as open a way as possible.

Finally in this section I want to consider a common misunderstanding of empathy and one that is sometimes used as a criticism of person-centred practitioners. This is the suggestion that empathy is 'identification with another' (Jacobs, 1988), and one that may lead to a kind of 'merging' – a common psychodynamic view of empathy. In fact, identification is most likely to be involved in sympathy rather than empathy. Whilst it is the case that we do use our own experiences to help us to get close to understanding others (it is the commonalities of human experiences that connect us after all), Rogers is clear in pointing out the importance of being aware of which emotions belong to whom and of being careful not to lose ourselves in the experiences of the other. He describes this as follows:

> 'being empathic, is to perceive the internal frame of reference of another with accuracy, and with the emotional components and meanings which pertain thereto, as if one were the other person, but without ever losing the "as if" condition. Thus it means to sense the hurt or the pleasure of another as he senses it, and to perceive the causes thereof as he perceives them, but without ever losing the recognition that it is *as if* I were hurt or pleased, etc. If this "as if" quality is lost, then the state is one of identification.' (1959, pp. 210–211)

The value of empathy

Empathy has many uses. In the world of business and commerce it is used in customer relations. Doctors are urged to use it because it improves compliance and therefore clinical outcomes. In therapy it can be used to encourage further exploration of issues and experiences, opening up new possibilities for the client and enabling greater self-understanding. However, to think in terms of the *uses* of empathy is akin to viewing it as a tool to achieve a goal. In these instances it is a *means to an end*. I prefer to think in terms of the *value* of empathy and to think of it as an *end in itself*, in which a person may feel recognised, understood, affirmed and validated (unconditional positive regard expressed through empathy) and connected. Rogers describes these values of empathy in the following way:

'To my mind, empathy is in itself a healing agent. It is one of the most potent aspects of therapy, because it releases, it confirms, it brings even the most frightened client into the human race. If a person can be understood, he or she belongs.' (1986, p. 129)

Yet perhaps to really know the value of empathy one has to experience receiving it.

Empathy in mental health settings

As psychiatry and mental health services have come to rely on and expect more from science and objective approaches, it becomes increasingly hard to make the case for person-centred empathy, the value and practice of which, in my observation, is fading ever more into the background as possibly a nice optional extra. Mental health professionals are taught to be detached and not to become emotionally involved in order, amongst other things, not to cloud objectivity. Empathy is often described as a 'soft skill' (at least in medical circles). Maybe then, it is only 'soft' doctors who advocate and practise it, unless, of course, it is for the scientific purpose of collecting data in order to evaluate, diagnose and pursue medical model goals. Thus, one of the major difficulties for developing person-centred empathy within mental health settings is that health care cultures neither recognise its value, nor support its development. There are too many other agendas, distractions and seemingly more important goals to pursue. Diagnoses result in stereotyping individuals, which is a major barrier to the openness of mind that is required to appreciate and empathise with a person's uniqueness. Given that the empathy I have described can also be intense and demanding, the realities of working in mental health settings are not generally conducive to adopting an empathic style of practice outside the context of therapy. It often simply seems too much effort.

Mental health settings also place particular demands on and challenges to empathy by virtue of the nature and degree of mental disturbance mental health professionals encounter. Given that empathy relies on having some common reference points with individuals, these may actually be few and far between when trying to understand the bizarre psychotic world of another. It can be harder to understand empathically people in the grip of severe mental disturbance and psychosis. However, trying to empathise here is, I believe, just as important as it is for people whose experiences are more easily understandable. In fact it is more important than ever to dissolve their sense of alienation and shame when this is their experience. It is important to understand and empathise with the fear, despair and isolation mental disturbance can engender.

As for empathising with a person's delusions or their despair, I think this is a highly skilled and demanding activity because it involves communicating understanding whilst not sharing (nor wanting to be perceived as agreeing with) his or her beliefs and feelings. Unfortunately, it is very easy for mental health professionals to be clumsy in their responses to such patients and I believe that such lack of care in communicating has led to the unfair accusation that empathy is a form of collusion and should therefore not be offered. Thus, poor communication can lead to a damaging misunderstanding of empathy, which in turn leads to a denouncement of its value in these instances. A potential opportunity to reduce a patient's sense of alienation has been turned into an occasion for increasing it. There is also an important debate here about whose reality matters. Avoidance of empathy towards psychotic experiences or profound despair clearly suggests that it is not patients' reality that matters.

One requirement of offering empathy though, is being secure enough in one's own sense of identity and strong enough in one's self not to get lost in the inner world of another, especially when that world is disturbed and confusing. I suspect that one of the major limitations for mental health professionals developing empathic understanding lies in the lack of attention to self-development. By self-development, I mean being committed to increasing self-awareness. This is not necessarily the same thing as gaining the required number of CPD (continuing professional development) points from attending courses. As for congruence and unconditional positive regard, self-awareness is a crucial ingredient for empathic understanding.

Conclusion

I hope I have demonstrated that congruence, unconditional positive regard and empathy constitute a powerful and healing set of attitudes and values, the expression of which involves far more than learning a set of communication skills or behavioural techniques. Yet, in my opinion, as the NHS becomes increasingly mechanised, cost and efficiency conscious, and as mental health professionals are expected to become more technically competent, develop more skills and to follow protocols and standardised care pathways, these essential attitudes and values are disappearing fast. I think this is a tragedy for patients and staff.

References

Borg M and Kristiansen K (2004) Recovery-oriented professionals: Helping relationships in mental health services. *Journal of Mental Health,* **13(5)**: 493–505.
Bozarth J (1998) *Person-Centred Therapy: A Revolutionary Paradigm.* PCCS Books, Ross-on-Wye.
Egan G (2004) *The Skilled Helper: a problem management and opportunity-development approach to helping* (7th edition). Brooks/Cole, Pacific Grove, California.
Embleton-Tudor L, Keemar K, Tudor K, Valentine J and Worrall M (2004) *The Person-Centred Approach. A Contemporary Introduction.* Palgrave Macmillan, Basingstoke.
Halpern J (2001) *From Detached Concern to Empathy. Humanizing Medical Practice.* Oxford University Press, Oxford.
Haugh S (2001) The Difficulties in the Conceptualisation of Congruence: A Way forward with Complexity Theory. In G Wyatt (ed) *Rogers' Therapeutic Conditions: Evolution, Theory and Practice, Volume 1. Congruence.* PCCS Books, Ross-on-Wye, pp. 116–130.
Jacobs M (1988) *Psychodynamic Counselling in Action.* Sage, London.
Lietaer G (2001a) Being Genuine as a Therapist: Congruence and Transparency. In G Wyatt (ed) *Rogers' Therapeutic Conditions: Evolution, Theory and Practice, Volume 1. Congruence.* PCCS Books, Ross-on-Wye, pp. 36–54.
Lietaer G (2001b) Unconditional Acceptance and Positive Regard. In J Bozarth and P Wilkins (eds) *Rogers' Therapeutic Conditions: Evolution, Theory and Practice, Volume 3. Unconditional Positive Regard.* PCCS Books, Ross-on-Wye, pp. 88–108.

McMillan M (2004) *The Person-centred approach to therapeutic change.* Sage, London.

Mearns D and Cooper M (2005) *Working at Relational Depth in Counselling and Psychotherapy.* Sage, London.

Mearns D and Thorne B (1999) *Person-Centred Counselling in Action* (2nd edition). Sage, London.

Mearns D and Thorne B (2000) *Person-Centred Therapy Today. New Frontiers in Theory and Practice.* Sage, London.

Oxford University Press (1996) *The Oxford English Reference Dictionary* (2nd edition). Oxford University Press, Oxford.

Purton C (2004) Focusing-oriented therapy. In P Sanders (ed) *The Tribes of the Person-Centred Nation: An introduction to the schools of therapy related to the Person-Centred Approach.* PCCS Books, Ross-on-Wye, pp. 45–66.

Rogers C (1957) The Necessary and Sufficient Conditions of Therapeutic Personality Change. *Journal of Consulting Psychology,* **21(2)**: 95–103.

Rogers C (1959) A theory of therapy, personality, and interpersonal relationships, as developed in the client-centred framework. In S Koch (ed) *Psychology: a study of a science. Study 1. Volume 3. Formulations of the person and the social context.* McGraw-Hill, New York, pp. 184–256.

Rogers C (1967) *On Becoming a Person. A therapist's view of psychotherapy.* Constable, London.

Rogers C (1980) *A Way of Being.* Houghton Mifflin, Boston, MA.

Rogers C (1986) Rogers, Kohut and Erickson: A personal perspective on some similarities and differences. *Person-Centred Review,* **1(2)**: 125–140.

Rogers C (1990) The Necessary and Sufficient Conditions of Therapeutic Personality Change. In H Kirschenbaum and V Land Henderson *The Carl Rogers Reader.* Constable, London, pp. 219–235. (Original work published in 1957)

Rogers C (1990) The Characteristics of a Helping Relationship. In H Kirschenbaum and V Land Henderson (eds) *The Carl Rogers Reader.* Constable, London, pp. 108–126. (Original work published 1958)

Rogers C (1990) A Client-centred/Person-centred Approach to Therapy. In H Kirschenbaum and V Land Henderson (eds) *The Carl Rogers Reader.* Constable, London, pp. 135–152. (Original work published 1986)

Rogers C (1995) What Understanding and Acceptance Mean to Me. *Journal of Humanistic Psychology,* **35(4)**: 7–22. (Transcript of a talk delivered in 1956).

Royal College of Psychiatrists (2000) *Good Psychiatric Practice.* Royal College of Psychiatrists, London.

Sims A (2003) *Symptoms in the Mind. An Introduction to Descriptive Psychopathology* (3rd edition). Saunders, London.

Spinelli E (2005) *The Interpreted World. An Introduction to Phenomenological Psychology* (2nd edition). Sage, London.

Thomas P (1997) *The Dialectics of Schizophrenia.* Free Association Books, London.

Tudor K and Worrall M (2006) *Person-Centred Therapy. A Clinical Philosophy.* Routledge, London.

Vincent S (2005) *Being Empathic. A companion for counsellors and therapists.* Radcliffe Publishing, Oxford.

Welwood J (2000) *Toward a Psychology of Awakening. Buddhism, Psychotherapy, and the Path of Personal and Spiritual Transformation.* Shambhala, Boston, MA.

Wilkins P (2001) Unconditional Positive Regard Reconsidered. In J Bozarth and P Wilkins (eds) *Rogers' Therapeutic Conditions: Evolution, Theory and Practice, Volume 3. Unconditional Positive Regard.* PCCS Books, Ross-on-Wye, pp. 35–48.

Worrall M (2001) Supervision and Empathic Understanding. In S Haugh and T Merry (eds) *Rogers' Therapeutic Conditions: Evolution, Theory and Practice, Volume 2. Empathy.* PCCS Books, Ross-on-Wye, pp. 206–217.

Chapter 9

The person-centred approach to severe psychopathology and psychosis

'The treatment of choice is to look for contact and work with that part of a person that is (still or already) rooted and operative, however small that part may be.'

(Van Werde, 2005, p. 166)

Introduction

In this chapter I aim to introduce the person-centred approach to more severe psychopathology and show that it is relevant to far more people with mental health needs than is often thought to be the case. I will challenge the view that the approach has limited applicability within secondary care mental health settings and is suitable only for the so-called 'worried well' generally seen in primary care settings.

In keeping with the general tendency of the person-centred approach not to be preoccupied with particular diagnostic categories, this chapter does not focus on specific illness categories. Instead, I shall concentrate on one important area of development of the person-centred approach that is directly relevant to a broad range of conditions. These are people for whom traditional psychotherapy is generally considered unsuitable. I refer here to individuals for whom the first of Rogers' conditions for constructive personality change, i.e. 'that two persons are in *contact*' (1959, p. 213), is difficult to meet. This chapter then, concerns contact (or 'psychological contact' as it is referred to in Rogers' 1957 paper) and a theory and practice that have been developed to work with individuals with so-called 'impaired contact'. They are people who have, for example, chronic psychotic disorders or dissociative states, or who have organic disease such as dementia or forms of brain damage.

I highlight this development of the person-centred approach because it is one area which has the potential to make a profound impact on much of psychiatric practice, both in residential and community care settings and within certain professional roles such as mental health nursing. This would of course require recognition of its value by policy-makers, managers, commissioners of mental health services and people in a position to influence the culture of mental health services. As I hope to show, adopting this approach to people who have impaired contact requires a major shift in attitudes towards the nature of mental health care – its goals and values.

What is 'psychological contact'?

This question is in fact very much open to debate. For me it taps into questions concerning the nature of conscious awareness (and by extension the concept of the unconscious), perception, how we *experience* other human beings, what it is we are experiencing, what is involved in such experiencing, and so on. I am particularly interested here though, in what Rogers has to say about it, although actually he says very little. He does not advance a theory of contact but describes it simply as each making 'some perceived difference in the experiential field of the other' (1957, p. 96). Even more simply, in the same section, he refers to it as a 'minimal relationship'.

What might Rogers mean by making some 'perceived difference in the experiential field of another'? He seems to suggest that persons are aware of each other and aware that they are making some difference to each other. Contact then, involves having an impact at some level. Interesting questions here concern whether or how much that awareness needs to be conscious. In fact Rogers also hypothesises that individuals may not be consciously aware of the impact of the other. He suggests that at some level even a catatonic patient may perceive someone's presence as making a difference. In this case, rather than using the term 'perception' of a difference in the experiential field, he uses the concept and term 'subception'. To subceive, according to Rogers, is when 'the organism can discriminate a stimulus and its meaning for the organism without utilizing the higher nerve centers involved in awareness' (1959, p. 200). In Rogers' terms then, experiences do not have to be symbolised in conscious awareness for the individual to be affected in some way by them. This suggests that our presence and actions have far more of an impact on those persons seemingly not consciously aware of us, such as people in catatonic states or even comas, than we usually assume.

However, is this 'minimal relationship' 'necessary and sufficient' for therapeutic personality change? Furthermore, can psychological contact be described as present or not, or are there degrees of contact? Within the person-centred community this latter question is very much open to debate, as discussed by Tudor and Worrall (2006), although Rogers clearly regards psychological contact as either present or not present. For him it is not a matter of degrees of contact, in contrast to the other conditions for therapeutic personality change, which he does regard as existing to varying degrees. As for whether a minimal relationship is necessary and sufficient, I need to remind myself that this is one (the first) of six conditions that together are described as 'necessary and sufficient'. Interestingly though, Rogers (1957) also describes it as more of a 'pre-condition' for therapy and that perhaps it should be set apart from the following five conditions.

It certainly makes sense to regard psychological contact as necessary for a therapeutic relationship (or therapy), but not necessarily for constructive personality change. Whether a relationship between two people is necessary for the occurrence of constructive personality change is a question Tudor and Worrall raise. They describe this with the following analogy: 'There are some tasks that require electricity, and some that we can achieve more efficiently or effectively with electricity. Electricity, however, is not the only source of power, and some of us, sometimes, cook with gas' (2006, p. 193). The conclusions I draw from this are that whilst psychological therapy or therapeutic relationships by definition require psychological contact to be made (the presence of a relationship), constructive personality change doesn't necessarily require psychological contact, although such change may be far more potent and effective in the context of relationship and psychological contact with another person. The type of change desired and needed is also an important consideration.

When contact is impaired: introducing 'pre-therapy'

Clearly, any conceptualisation of 'impaired contact' requires a conceptualisation of what contact is and consists of, about which, as highlighted above, Rogers says very little. One of the reasons Rogers does not develop a theory of contact is probably because, as Van Werde (2002a) points out, it was simply a 'given' for most of the clients he worked with. In other words, because he worked with people in therapy, as a therapist, contact could be assumed.

However, there are many people for whom therapy is neither considered nor offered. These are people usually with more severe psychopathology for whom establishing psychological contact and the capacity to either make or sustain relationship is in question. Fortunately, this is an area which person-centred theorists and practitioners working in mental health or other health settings have since developed. In particular I refer to the pioneering work of an American psychologist, Garry Prouty, who has developed what is termed 'pre-therapy'. Pre-therapy evolved through Prouty's search for a way of helping those patient/client populations who 'cannot fully use relationship or Experiencing processes' (Prouty, 2002a, p. 55), drawing upon his experience of working with people with chronic psychosis, schizophrenia and learning disabilities. It was not developed specifically as a precursor for therapy as the term 'pre-therapy' suggests. However, pre-therapy techniques can facilitate the establishment of a relationship, or psychological contact, such that therapy can then helpfully be offered to some people. Pre-therapy can be considered a specific application of the person-centred approach. It consists of a specific method built upon a theory of contact and reflects the broad philosophical principles of the person-centred approach. What follows describes a theory of contact as proposed by Prouty, after which I shall describe its practical application.

Contact functions

Prouty's theory of psychological contact draws on phenomenological perspectives. This is to say that it draws upon the philosophy of how we experience phenomena. The phenomena with which we are in contact Prouty separates into *reality, others* and *self*. Contact then comes to be understood as contact with reality (the world: an awareness of people, places, things and events); with other people (the ability to communicate and give 'meaningful expression of our perceived world and self to others' (Prouty, 2002a, p. 59)); and with our affective self (which Prouty describes as an awareness of our moods, feelings and emotions in response to the world). Contact then, is a broad concept that describes internal psychological functions enabling us to be 'in touch' with the world around us, other people and ourselves, hence Prouty's term 'contact functions'.

Impaired contact thus refers to a loss or impairment of contact functions such that awareness of reality, the self and others and the ability to communicate awareness, are disturbed. However, rather than seeing this in deficiency terms, Prouty views such impairment in terms of a *potential* to experience and express experience. The central construct he uses here is that of the 'Pre-Expressive Self' which he describes as 'a *meta-psychological* concept that refers to the propensity, for the yet to be integrated experience, to form expression' (2002b, p. 20, original italics). In other words, contact functions can be seen in terms of their potential to be developed. The pre-expressive self can become expressive, in the right conditions, although whether all people with impaired contact can become expressive is doubtful in my view. I am thinking here of people with organic conditions such as brain damage or dementia. Nevertheless, I do believe that the potential to develop expression or restore contact functions is often ignored or neglected in health care settings and that the potential for development is much greater than we often assume is the case.

Before leaving this section I would like to draw attention to one area of possible confusion when referring to the term 'contact'. Being 'out of touch with reality', or having 'lost contact with reality' is often how mental health professionals describe psychosis. From what I have said about contact and relationship so far in this chapter, the logical and simplistic conclusion from this is that psychosis prevents relationship and therefore therapy or therapeutic relating. This is clearly not the case because many people with psychotic experiences such as hallucinations or delusions are able to communicate and express themselves very effectively, as well as being in touch with considerable portions of reality and their affective selves. Psychosis is not necessarily a barrier to relationship or therapy, although sometimes it can be, particularly when severe (severe here could describe both acute and chronic conditions). The common description of psychosis as representing a state of having lost contact with reality (which raises questions about what we mean by reality) does not relate to the forms of impaired contact with which pre-therapy is generally concerned. In addition, pre-therapy is not exclusively applicable to people with psychosis, although it was originally developed largely with this patient population in mind.

Making contact: the method of pre-therapy

The method of pre-therapy aims to develop or restore the contact functions previously described. It involves a set of simple techniques, which are grounded in person-centred attitudes such as unconditional positive regard. In fact Prouty states that 'Pre-Therapy cannot be undertaken without the attitude of unconditional positive regard' (2001a, p. 82). Prouty also describes pre-therapy as a 'new mode of empathy' (2001b, p. 155). In addition, whilst pre-therapy is a set of techniques, their skilful application could be considered an art. They are not to be practised in a mechanical way but involve an attempt to tune in to a person's individual and unique world. The non-directive attitude is also a facet of pre-therapy because of the desire to follow the patient's expression and process.

Contact reflections: a form of empathy

When Rogers describes the six conditions for constructive personality change, he refers to empathy as follows: 'the therapist is *experiencing* an *empathic*

Severe psychopathology and psychosis **153**

understanding of the client's *internal frame of reference'* (1959, p. 213, original italics). However, given the difficulties of sensing, let alone understanding, the frame of reference of someone who is very disturbed, perhaps with the thought disorder or delusions of severe psychosis or the withdrawal of severe depression, it is necessary to find a way of communicating that is different from the more usual empathic understanding responses. The more usual forms of empathic understanding and expression can rely on abstraction, the use of metaphor, symbols and essences of meaning. In contrast, Prouty describes the empathic approach of pre-therapy as 'an extraordinary literal and concrete form of empathic response' (2001b, p. 158). Pre-therapy empathic responses to patients are concrete reflections of their behaviours. (They are, in fact, particularly empathic towards individuals with concrete ways of experiencing reality.)

The concreteness of 'contact reflections', as they are termed, is best demonstrated with examples which I will now give, as I describe the five types of contact reflections pre-therapy describes. *Situational reflections* ('*SR*') concern the person and their environment with the aim of encouraging contact with reality. Examples might be such things as saying 'You are looking out of the window' or 'I am sitting by your side'. *Facial reflections* ('*FR*') help to develop affective contact and involve observations of facial expression such as 'You are frowning' (not, incidentally, 'You look cross' or 'puzzled' which would involve an evaluation, and which therefore is not phenomenological). *Body reflections* ('*BR*') can either take the form of duplicating the patient's body movement such as copying them as they place their hand on their head, or it can be a verbal description of movement or body position such as 'You are standing on one leg'. *Word-for-word reflections* ('*WWR*') aim to develop communicative contact by reflecting (repeating) portions of a patient's speech, particularly word or sentence fragments of the generally incoherent speech of people with gross thought disorder. Finally, *reiterative reflections* ('*RR*') are simply a reiteration of reflections that led to a response and are a way of attempting re-contact. They are based on the principle of repeating what works.

The empathy of pre-therapy, then, is towards pre-expressive behaviours rather than on understanding a person's frame of reference. It aims to provide patients 'with a "web of contact" at different levels, thus allowing ... opportunities of expression and relatedness' (Prouty, 2002b, p. 17).

It is by no means easy for mental health professionals or person-centred therapists to make the transition from the abstract to the concrete and it is this that makes pre-therapy a more skilful approach than it might at first appear. Another impediment to using concrete reflections is fearing that they may sound, or be perceived as, condescending, as Sommerbeck (2003) experiences when she starts to use pre-therapy with patients in a psychiatric hospital. However, she comes to experience the reflections 'as a gentle expression of my wish to get in contact with them' (2003, p. 72). Keeping focus on the goal of establishing contact should prevent being overly anxious about getting the technique right or about how the reflections sound. Sommerbeck also provides some vignettes of her experiences of using pre-therapy, especially with patients who seem to move in and out of contact and who require the mental health professional or therapist to move flexibly back and forth between concrete contact reflections and the more usual empathic understanding responses.

Vignettes

I now provide two vignettes to give a flavour of using pre-therapy, although it needs to be borne in mind that, according to Van Werde, 'when speaking about Pre-Therapy, and especially when reflections are written down, they tend to look simplistic, mechanical and a mere act of repeating. Beautiful moments of delicate interaction, receptiveness for the existential situation, the necessary discipline and concentration, and the relatively distant playfulness combined with a sincere and close compassion are hard to transfer on to paper' (2002b, p. 63).

The first is an incident described by Prouty. I have chosen this example because it demonstrates a situation in which mental health professionals may be tempted to use tranquillising medication to control a potential crisis situation, where pre-therapy techniques may well be as, if not more, effective. Throughout the transcript the types of contact reflections used are indicated.

'The client was one of seven on an outing from a half-way house. She was seated in the rear seat of the van. As I looked in the rear-view mirror, I observed the client crouched down into the seat with one arm outstretched above her head. The client's face was filled with terror and her voice began to escalate in screams. I pulled the van off the road and asked the volunteer to take the others out of the van. I sat next to the client, sharing the same fear.

CLIENT:	[In rising voice.] It's pulling me in.
THERAPIST:	[WWR] It's pulling me in.
CLIENT:	[Continuing to slip further down into the seat, with left arm outstretched. Eyes still closed.]
THERAPIST:	[BR] Your body is slipping down into the seat. Your arm is in the air.
THERAPIST:	[SR] We are in the van. You are sitting next to me.
CLIENT:	[Screaming.]
THERAPIST:	[FR] You are screaming, Carol.
CLIENT:	It's pulling me in.
THERAPIST:	[WWR] It's pulling you in.
THERAPIST:	[SR] Carol, we are in the van. You are sitting next to me.
THERAPIST:	[FR] Something is frightening you. You are screaming.
CLIENT:	[Patient screaming.] It's sucking me in.
THERAPIST:	[WWR] It's sucking you in.
THERAPIST:	[SR/BR] We are in the van, Carol. You are sitting next to me. Your arm is in the air.
CLIENT:	[Beginning to sob very hard. Arms dropped to lap.] It was the vacuum cleaner.
THERAPIST:	[WWR] It was the vacuum cleaner.
CLIENT:	[Direct eye contact.] She did it with the vacuum cleaner. [Continued in a normal tone of voice.] I thought it was gone. She used to turn on the vacuum cleaner when I was bad and put the hose right on my arm. I thought it sucked it in. [Less sobbing. It should be noted that daily this patient would kiss her arm up to her elbow and stroke it continually.]

THERAPIST: [*WWR*] Your arm is still here. It didn't get sucked into the
                       vacuum cleaner.
CLIENT: [Smiled and was held by therapist.]

Later that afternoon, a psychotherapy session was held and the client began
to delve into her feelings about punishment received as a child. The kissing
and stroking of the arm ceased. This vignette illustrates how the client was
helped to deal with the acute episode in a psychologically beneficial manner
without medications. The client was able to experience how her symptoms
of arm kissing and stroking related to a negative childhood emotional trauma
of her mother threatening her with a vacuum cleaner. In addition, the client
was able to use this newly integrated material as a basis for further therapy
concerning her mother.' (Prouty, 2002c, pp. 68–9).*

* With thanks to PCCS Books for kind permission to reproduce this extract.

The following vignette is described by Dion Van Werde, a person-centred
psychologist working in a psychiatric hospital in Belgium. He illustrates the
difficulty of knowing whether the patient is communicating from a psychotic
state or not.

'The client, Marianne, walked into the nurses' office and said "Are they
coming to get me?" In that moment I did not know whether psychotic
(paranoid) content was being expressed, whether this was congruent, reality-
based communication, or maybe even both. This particular level of functioning I elsewhere call grey-zone functioning (Van Werde, 2002a, b). Marianne
had been with us for two weeks and I knew that psychosis was never far
away. On the other hand, most of the time, congruent communication was
possible. So, I was faced with the problem of how to respond to this question.
Since reacting to a client always involves a decision, or at least retro-
spectively we should be able to construct which elements played a role in our
decision, I shall share with you what went through my mind and how things
proceeded. The mere doubt about her level of functioning (psychotic and/or
congruent) made me choose to respond with contact reflections.

DION: [*WWR*] Are they coming to get me?
               [Since Marianne did not react verbally, but kept staring at me
               with an unchanged body posture, I tried again to bring her
               into contact with what was actually happening.]
               [*SR/RR*] You look at me and ask if they are coming to get you.
MARIANNE: Are they coming to get me?
               [This strengthened my hypothesis that she was in a psychotic
               state, so I reflected what she did with her body as an extra
               means for anchorage.]
DION: [*BR/RR*] Just a second ago you looked up
               [and I myself looked at the window in the same way that
               she had], and asked "Are they coming to get me?"
MARIANNE: I always hear airplanes and things.
               [Obviously she was now showing something of her psychotic
               world. I maintained eye contact and reflected.]

DION: [*WWR*] I always hear airplanes and things.
MARIANNE: What do you think? … I want to know.
                   [I was not clear what she meant by this question. Was she
                   asking my opinion about the situation, the interaction or
                   about airplanes? Does she mean that these things are going to
                   take her away? In that moment I myself experienced the
                   blend of the two worlds: the reality of our conversation and/
                   or the reality of her paranoid psychotic system. All I felt I
                   could do was to reflect her question and hope that she would
                   clarify it to herself and to me.]
DION: [*WWR*] You ask me what I think.
MARIANNE: Are they coming to get me?
                   [I had a very clear feeling that every word was important but I
                   did not know what she was going through or where these
                   words were leading her. I carefully reflected only what she
                   had given thus making sure not to distract her from her
                   own process.]
DION: [*WWR*] Are they coming to get me? Just a while ago you said
                   "I always hear airplanes and things" [*RR*]. Now you are look-
                   ing at me [*SR*] and ask: "Are they coming to get me?" [*WWR*].
MARIANNE: Can I phone home?
                   [This was a direct question and I gave a congruent answer
                   since I thought that her level of functioning was more
                   congruent and contact reflections were no longer indicated,
                   so I replied.]
DION: You already phoned home: what did you agree with them?
MARIANNE: They are coming at 2pm. It's still one and a half hours to wait.
                   [This was obviously Reality Contact. Her parents were going
                   to pick her up for a weekend leave at 2pm and it was indeed
                   only 12.30pm. I continued on a congruent level and made
                   some suggestions.]
DION: Indeed, so what will you do? Perhaps walk around a bit?
                   Perhaps you could lay down on your bed …?
MARIANNE: Not on my bed, otherwise I think they will come and get me.
                   I'm not sure I would survive.
                   [Probably my suggestions have induced her to become more
                   psychotic once again, so I returned to Word-for Word Reflec-
                   tion and tried not to go beyond what she gave me since her
                   anchorage was fragile.]
DION: [*WWR*] You don't know if you would survive. [*RR*] You say:
                   "I'm not going to lay down, otherwise I think they will come
                   and get me."
MARIANNE: I don't know if I will be alive.
DION: [*SR*] You look at me and say: "I don't know if I will be alive."
                   [*WWR*] Your eyes look sad. [*FR*] You shiver. [*BR*]
MARIANNE: I don't feel easy at all.

In this last statement Marianne has contacted her feelings. This is Affective
Contact. In the interaction that followed, Marianne very adequately talked

about her fear of travelling, made a phone call to change the hour of pick-up and empathically understood her mother who tried to reassure her daughter about the pick-up.

This dialogue illustrates the thinking of the practitioner using client-centred pre-therapy methodology in everyday contact with patients. Marianne was helped to change her level of functioning in such a way as to make more contact with her feelings and with the shared reality. This step was made possible through empathic contact with Marianne at the level on which she was functioning and with respect for her own tempo.' (Van Werde, 2003, pp. 126–28).*

*With thanks to Sage for kind permission to reproduce this extract.

The value and uses of pre-therapy

Pre-therapy is an established method of trying to restore or strengthen the contact functions of people with impaired contact, whatever the cause of that impairment. Its value can be expressed in terms of behavioural change and Prouty has also developed the concept of 'contact behaviours', which he describes as the 'operationalised aspect of psychological contact', along with developing ways of measuring behaviours (Prouty, 2002a, p. 60). Demonstrable change in contact behaviours include increased social and occupational functioning, increased self-expression such as expression of needs and increased opportunities for psychosocial intervention.

However, the value of pre-therapy techniques can also be viewed in terms of establishing connection and relationship with people at high risk of experiencing isolation and alienation. Whilst on one level it does seek to effect change, when practised in the spirit of the person-centred approach, e.g. with the attitude of unconditional positive regard, it is a way of validating a person's experience and seeing such experience as meaningful, even if not understandable. As Van Werde points out, 'in person-centred working it is much more important to be psychologically "present" and in "contact" with the client than actually to understand what the client is communicating' (2003, p. 124). Thus, practising pre-therapy techniques, underpinned by the philosophy of the person-centred approach, will be a way of being alongside someone rather than understanding them. It will be as much about seeing the value of relating at a basic existential level – indeed, simply valuing relatedness and connection – as it is about trying to develop contact functions. This does create a tension between doing and being. Recognising this, Van Werde writes, 'following the experiential process of the client on the one hand and offering and working with the shared reality on the other. That is to say, we hold the tension between "being with the client" and "doing with the client"' (1998, p. 207). He does not, though, see these two aspects of pre-therapy as being in opposition to each other.

When thinking about the sorts of client and patient populations for which pre-therapy may be applicable, its value and uses extend beyond the mental health settings with which this book is concerned. As highlighted at the beginning of this chapter, impaired contact may be a feature of a broad range of conditions. Pre-therapy has been used across this range and some of this work is documented in the literature. Prouty (1994; 2002b) describes the practice of pre-therapy with people with chronic psychosis and learning disabilities. Van Werde (2002b; 2005) has developed the practice of pre-therapy in more acute psychiatric settings, particularly in creating a ward culture (or 'contact milieu') that regularly uses pre-therapy techniques. Roy (1991) has practised pre-therapy with people experiencing the dissociation of multiple personality disorder and Coffeng (1996; 2002) describes working with people who have experienced trauma and also dissociation. This method of working has also been used with people with dementia (Van Werde and Morton, 1999; Dodds, Morton and Prouty, 2004) where the emphasis is more on being alongside individuals.

One of the other valuable aspects of this way of working is that it can be used by all members of staff, across all professions, and not just those with professional qualifications. Pre-therapy can be used by in-patient staff, community mental health teams, crisis teams, Care Trust workers within the NHS, within nursing and residential homes and Special Needs schools. It can also be used by family members and carers of people whose contact is impaired. Catherine Clarke in the UK has written about her experiences of using pre-therapy techniques with her son (2005a; 2005b) and shows how practising pre-therapy techniques benefits both the relative being cared for and the carer too.

Current developments and future possibilities

In the UK efforts are currently being made to introduce pre-therapy into mental health nurse training and also into dementia care (see useful website addresses at the end of this chapter for further details), but in general this way of working is as yet little known in the NHS. Developments of the approach have occurred predominantly in mainland Europe, particularly in Belgium and The Netherlands, but also in Italy and Germany. An international network has also now been in existence for several years. An overview of pre-therapy developments in Europe is provided by Prouty, Van Werde and Pörtner (2002).

Perhaps the most notable development has been the creation of a ward culture in a psychiatric hospital in Ghent, Belgium, in which staff have been trained to use pre-therapy techniques. The development of this 'contact milieu' has been pioneered by Dion Van Werde, who writes about anchorage as a core concept when working with people who experience psychosis (1998). Van Werde is not naïve to the challenges of integrating pre-therapy into mental health secondary care settings. For him understanding the system and managerial and political realities is crucial. He acknowledges the limitations of resources, the use of medication and the importance of fitting into the requirements of the organisation.

Introducing the approach to mental health professionals presents many challenges since it requires a shift in the mindset of how patients are responded to and perhaps a re-conceptualisation of the nature of mental disturbance. For example, rather than seeing psychotic symptoms as the main problem, Van Werde (2002b) sees the problem as an imbalance between healthy and problematic functioning which leads to the goal of strengthening the healthy part rather than automatically trying to eradicate the symptoms.

It is hard to imagine being able to create a similar ward culture here in the UK, particularly at a time when the government and mental health services are restructuring and cutting services to recoup large debts. Short-term financial considerations are one of the greatest impediments to developing pre-therapy as a valuable approach that mental health professionals can use. The required focus on targets, outcome measures and increasingly mechanistic and standardised ways of working with patients, with their associated bureaucratic burdens, creates a culture in which simply connecting with people and being alongside them are neither valued nor prioritised. One of the most common approaches to 'managing' patients, particularly in hospital, is to prescribe medication and essentially wait for it to take effect. An approach that is based on person-centred philosophy and attitudes is likely to be resisted in a culture that is obsessed with quantifying outcomes and evidenced-based practice. For Pörtner, 'What we need is a broad, holistic, long-term view that does not observe each task and the time it takes isolated from the context. A concept emphasising the well-being and individuality of the persons cared for, and at the same time allowing the staff to experience their work as useful and satisfying, a concept fostering and making use of the resources of all the people involved, in the long term will probably even save time and money' (2002, p. 173). I agree, although I am currently pessimistic about the ability of our Department of Health to take the 'broad, holistic, long-term view' required.

Where I am more optimistic though, concerns the potential for pre-therapy to be used by professionals and by carers and family members in the community and for those benefits to make themselves known, with the possibility of a gradual influencing of the culture of mental health care and challenge to traditional practices. At present, in the UK, I think the greatest opportunity for promoting the value of pre-therapy probably lies within the non-statutory sector and user and carer organisations.

References

Clarke C (2005a) A Carer's Experience of the Mental Health System. In S Joseph and R Worsley (eds) *Person-Centred Psychopathology: A positive psychology of mental health.* PCCS Books, Ross-on-Wye, pp. 9–20.

Clarke C (2005b) Prouty's contact work: a carer's perspective. *Mental Health Practice,* **9(1)**: 24–27.

Coffeng T (1996) The delicate approach to early trauma. In R Hutterer, G Pawlowsky, P Schmid and R Stipsis (eds) *Client-centred and Experiential Psychotherapy: A Paradigm in Motion.* Peter Lang, Frankfurt am Main, pp. 481–493.

Coffeng T (2002) Contact in the Therapy of Trauma and Dissociation. In G Wyatt and P Sanders (eds) *Rogers' Therapeutic Conditions: Evolution, Theory and Practice, Volume 4. Contact and Perception.* PCCS Books, Ross-on-Wye, pp. 153–167.

Dodds P, Morton I and Prouty G (2004) Using pre-therapy techniques in dementia care. *Journal of Dementia Care,* **12(2)**: 25–28.

Pörtner M (2002) Pre-Therapy in Europe. In G Prouty, D Van Werde and M Pörtner *Pre-Therapy. Reaching contact-impaired clients.* PCCS Books, Ross-on-Wye, pp. 121–177.

Prouty G (1994) *Theoretical Evolutions in Person-centered/Experiential Therapy: Applications to schizophrenic and retarded psychosis.* Praeger, New York.

Prouty G (2001a) Unconditional Positive Regard and Pre-Therapy: An Exploration. In J Bozarth and P Wilkins (eds) *Rogers' Therapeutic Conditions: Evolution, Theory and Practice, Volume 3. Unconditional Positive Regard.* PCCS Books, Ross-on-Wye, pp. 76–87.

Prouty G (2001b) A New Mode of Empathy: Empathic contact. In S Haugh and T Merry (eds) *Rogers' Therapeutic Conditions: Evolution, Theory and Practice, Volume 2. Empathy.* PCCS Books, Ross-on-Wye, pp. 155–162.

Prouty G (2002a) Pre-Therapy as a Theoretical System. In G Wyatt and P Sanders (eds) *Rogers' Therapeutic Conditions: Evolution, Theory and Practice, Volume 4. Contact and Perception.* PCCS Books, Ross-on-Wye, pp. 54–62.

Prouty G (2002b) The Foundations of Pre-Therapy. In G Prouty, D Van Werde and M Pörtner *Pre-Therapy. Reaching contact-impaired clients.* PCCS Books, Ross-on-Wye, pp. 1–60.

Prouty G (2002c) The Practice of Pre-Therapy. In G Wyatt and P Sanders (eds) *Rogers' Therapeutic Conditions: Evolution, Theory and Practice, Volume 4. Contact and Perception.* PCCS Books, Ross-on-Wye, pp. 63–75.

Prouty G, Van Werde D and Pörtner M (2002) *Pre-Therapy. Reaching contact-impaired clients.* PCCS Books, Ross-on-Wye.

Rogers C (1957) The Necessary and Sufficient Conditions of Therapeutic Personality Change. *Journal of Consulting Psychology,* **21(2)**: 25–103.

Rogers C (1959) A theory of therapy, personality, and interpersonal relationships, as developed in the client-centered framework. In S Koch (ed) *Psychology: a study of a science. Study 1. Volume 3. Formulations of the person and the social context.* McGraw-Hill, New York, pp. 184–256.

Roy B (1991) A client-centered approach to multiple personality and dissociated process. In L Fusek (ed) *New Directions in Client-Centered Therapy: Practice with Difficult Populations.* Chicago Counselling and Psychotherapy Research Center, Chicago, pp. 18–40.

Sommerbeck L (2003) *The Client-Centred Therapist in Psychiatric Contexts. A therapists' guide to the psychiatric landscape and its inhabitants.* PCCS Books, Ross-on-Wye.

Tudor K and Worral M (2006) *Person-Centred Therapy. A Clinical Philosophy.* Routledge, London.

Van Werde D (1998) 'Anchorage' as a Core Concept in Working with Psychotic People. In B Thorne and E Lambers (eds) *Person-Centred Therapy. A European Perspective.* Sage, London.

Van Werde D (2002a) Prouty's Pre-Therapy and Contact-work with a Broad Range of Persons' Pre-expressive Functioning. In G Wyatt and P Sanders (eds) *Rogers' Therapeutic Conditions: Evolution, Theory and Practice, Volume 4. Contact and Perception.* PCCS Books, Ross-on-Wye, pp. 168–181.

Van Werde D (2002b) Pre-Therapy Applied on a Psychiatric Ward. In G Prouty, D Van Werde and M Pörtner *Pre-Therapy. Reaching contact-impaired clients.* PCCS Books, Ross-on-Wye, pp. 61–120.

Van Werde D (2003) Dealing with the possibility of psychotic content in a seemingly congruent communication. In D Mearns *Developing Person-Centred Counselling* (2nd edition). Sage, London.

Van Werde D (2005) Facing Psychotic Functioning: Person-centred contact work in residential psychiatric care. In S Joseph and R Worsley (eds) *Person-Centred Psychopathology: A Positive Psychology of Mental Health.* PCCS Books, Ross-on-Wye, pp. 158–168.

Van Werde D and Morton I (1999) The Relevance of Prouty's Pre-Therapy to Dementia Care. In I Morton *Person-Centred Approaches to Dementia Care.* Winslow Press, Bicester, Oxon, pp. 139–166.

Further reading

- Prouty G, Van Werde D and Pörtner M (2002) *Pre-Therapy. Reaching contact-impaired clients.* PCCS Books, Ross-on-Wye. This is a good introduction to pre-therapy and includes many vignettes.

- Sommerbeck L (2003) *The Client-Centred Therapist in Psychiatric Contexts. A therapists' guide to the psychiatric landscape and its inhabitants.* PCCS Books, Ross-on-Wye. This book also offers an introduction to pre-therapy and particularly how it is used by a person-centred therapist working in a psychiatric hospital, exploring the numerous tensions and dilemmas this involves. Sommerbeck also illustrates pre-therapy with vignettes.
- Two useful website addresses are:
  – www.psychological-wellbeing.co.uk provides some general information on pre-therapy.
  – www.pretherapy.com is the website for the Pre-Therapy International Network, although it only provides a list of contacts and references.

Chapter 10

Looking after ourselves: support, supervision and personal development

'Mental health services are *human* services – services are provided and received by people in relationship with one another. ... Receiving support and feeling supported make the difference between thriving and surviving in work that is often intensely personally demanding.'

(Gilbert, 2004, p. 164)

Introduction

Ten years ago I wrote a short article entitled 'How much do we matter?' for a doctors' magazine (Freeth, 1996). Motivated by a sense of outrage, I wrote this article to highlight the 'unjust, insensitive and short-sighted institution' that I perceived the NHS to be regarding the needs of staff. It was my experience that the strong message given to health professionals working in the NHS is that we did not matter – we were simply commodities to be used, moved around and discarded. I believe, sadly, that little has changed. In fact, there is now abundant evidence (for example, in the health care and medical press) of significant decline in staff morale over the past ten years. Despite statements from politicians and senior managers praising staff for the 'fantastic' work we do, the realities of working in the NHS suggest to me that these messages are at best superficial and at worst hollow and cynical. Furthermore, there appears no light at the end of the tunnel as the Labour government continues to accelerate the pace of reform of public services, believing that getting the economics and financial structures right far outweighs the importance of the health, well-being and levels of motivation of health professionals.

Looking after ourselves is the theme of this final chapter. However, it focuses not only on matters of health and well-being, but also on our professional and personal development, which is a crucial foundation of mental health practice. The process of supervision forms a large part of this discussion. In particular, I highlight a person-centred approach to supervision, drawing upon my own experience of receiving person-centred supervision and how this enables me to bring the person-centred approach into my work as a mental health professional. To begin with though, I draw attention to the particular stresses and hazards of being a mental health professional. To be aware of these stresses enables greater awareness of our personal and professional needs.

The hazards of being a mental health professional

'Burnout' has become an increasingly recognised phenomenon amongst health professionals. Characteristics of burnout include emotional exhaustion, disillusionment, detachment, reduced energy, negative job attitudes and reduced care and concern for others (Roberts, 2000). I have certainly witnessed its effects on a significant proportion of the mental health workforce across all the various professions and have experienced some of its features myself. Maybe I have been fortunate to have experienced this early enough in my working life to realise the importance of giving myself various career options. In considering carefully my options I have attempted to minimise the risk of experiencing the end stage of a burning out process that seems to have afflicted so many of my NHS colleagues further on in their careers when it is perhaps less easy to change the course and pattern of their working lives.

For numerous reasons the mental health workforce seem to be at particular risk of experiencing burnout. Similarly, according to Adshead, 'working in mental health seems (both predictably and ironically) to be especially hazardous for the mental health of psychiatric staff' (2005, p. 331). And if not risking mental illness or burnout, we are certainly at risk of experiencing high levels of work-related stress, with the various consequences of this, for example, its damaging effects on family and home life. This is why the topic of looking after ourselves deserves critical attention.

It is not hard to explore the sources of stress when working in mental health services. In thinking about these, those factors connected to the nature of the work, particularly the psychological demands of working with mentally and emotionally disturbed people, are especially significant. Another category of factors relates to working within the particular system and organisation. A further category of stress concerns our perceived role within society and the unreasonable expectations placed upon mental health professionals, particularly in the face of social and societal problems. For example, I find it stressful responding to expectations that my job should concern public protection over and above a therapeutic role of providing care. Another major source of stress for me is when I experience a conflict of expectations and values, particularly when my values clash with those of the organisation and policy makers. As someone who tries to work according to person-centred values and philosophy within a culture in which these values are rarely recognised, or recognised but sidelined, I need to be aware of the impact on me of this on-going conflict and source of stress. Needless to say, lack of control over workload, unremitting demands, major organisational and often badly managed change, limited resources to provide quality care (often in the form of staff shortages), ambiguity around roles and responsibilities of mental health professionals, lack of recognition of the needs of staff, feelings of powerlessness and fear of blame, criticism and being scapegoated, are all ready sources of stress falling into one or more of the above categories.

As well as external sources of stress, there may well be for many of us internal factors that make us more vulnerable. In a review of the literature addressing various explanations for the hypothesis that mental health staff are at higher risk of mental distress and illness, Walsh and Walsh (2001) consider 'individual vulnerability factors' and the suggestion that people who are themselves vulnerable to psychological stress or who have experienced mental illness are attracted to working in the mental health professions. Research on this is limited, although this doesn't imply that there is no truth in this suggestion. However, there is currently more evidence that mental health staff 'experience distinctive working conditions that may be psychologically hazardous' (p. 126).

Whatever formal research findings may or may not reveal, certainly anecdotally the concept of the 'wounded healer' resonates with many mental health professionals. It is not hard to find literature in which mental health professionals talk about their experiences of mental illness. One of the best-known examples is a book edited by Rippere and Williams (1985) entitled 'Wounded Healers. Mental Health Workers' Experiences of Depression'. The American psychologist and professor of psychiatry Kay Redfield Jamison is well-known for her account of her experience of living and working with a manic-depressive illness in her highly acclaimed book 'An Unquiet Mind' (1995). Nevertheless, in the UK at least, it is still not easy for mental health professionals to talk about their vulnerabilities or experiences of mental distress. In the medical profession there is what has been described as a 'conspiracy of silence and denial' (Ghodse, 2000, p. 10). Ghodse describes how doctors are afraid of admitting their health needs, particularly mental health needs and, for example, symptoms of depression and anxiety. There is a tendency for doctors to perceive their health problems and needs as a sign of personal failure, and/or a threat to their livelihoods. Barker *et al* (1998) also describe how mental health nurses have a fear of 'coming out' about their experiences of mental ill health and fear how doing so might adversely affect career progression.

The 'wounded healer'

The concept of the 'wounded healer' is actually a creative and positive one, and, as Barker *et al* (1998) suggest, it is well established in Western medicine. Within this concept, there is a valuing of the wound or vulnerability that may, amongst other things, enhance empathic understanding and lead to more compassionate and insightful helping professionals. However, learning to appreciate our woundedness and vulnerabilities is a process many mental health professionals, in my experience, find hard to do. Unfortunately, all too often there is a 'them' and 'us' mentality within mental health organisations, in which the idea that we all belong to the same human family with the same frailties and vulnerabilities, albeit expressed in different ways, is resisted. There is often a tendency to regard the 'mentally ill' and 'mad' as 'them', perhaps as a way of protecting ourselves either from our own fears of mental illness or from feelings of shame concerning our vulnerabilities and weaknesses. Without adequate recognition of wounds what can be a rich source of empathy, therapeutic relating and effective caring, can also potentially be disastrous for patients as well as for the mental health professional. If he or she is not a liability then at the very least his or her caring work and relationships may simply be of limited quality and effectiveness. Recognition is the key, and Barker *et al*, when writing about mental health nurses, argue that their use of their experiences of mental distress needs to be 'developed carefully, arguably within the context of sensitive clinical supervision' (1998, p. 337). It is the topic of supervision to which I now turn.

Supervision within mental health settings

One of the conclusions Walsh and Walsh draw in their paper on the health of the mental health workforce is that 'this group warrant special attention if they are to maintain their mental health and provide services of an acceptable quality' (2001, p. 126). They also suggest that further research is necessary to clarify the nature of this special attention.

Supervision is one way of attending to the needs of the mental health workforce. However, although I argue for the importance of high quality, readily available supervision for all mental health professionals, whatever their profession, level of expertise and experience, it is only one factor in the equation when considering the stress levels and needs of staff, and it is only one form of support. Supervision may help to strengthen the foundations, but if unreasonable and excessive loads continue to be piled on, even the strongest foundations will eventually crack. Thus, another vital part of supporting mental health professionals is to recognise the pressures and stresses they are under, seek to keep them within reasonable and manageable proportions and, likewise, have realistic expectations of them. This should be a key task of managers, politicians and policy makers but it is unfortunately one that many consistently fail to recognise as important. It is simply not in their field of vision. However good supervision arrangements may be, if a person's job is damaging to their health, due to organisational factors for example, the only solution may be to remove him or herself entirely from the equation. I say this to make the point that supervision can only achieve so much. Other forms of support are also usually necessary, both of a formal and informal nature. Even then, it may not be enough to mitigate the effects of working in environments that are potentially damaging. Nevertheless, good quality, regular supervision can be invaluable, although, I would suggest, currently rare in the NHS.

There are many different perspectives on supervision and because of this there is no overarching definition, although various descriptions highlight the process, goals, tasks (functions) and relationships (roles) of supervision. Tudor and Worrall (2004a), who have reviewed the generic literature on supervision, note various aspects of it that have emerged and been expanded upon over the years. The topics they identify include the functions of supervision, the process of supervision, development in supervision, how supervision is organised, its context and the roles of the supervisor and supervisee.

The purposes and tasks of supervision

One of the initial key tasks is to agree at the outset the purposes and tasks (the latter sometimes described as functions, although their meaning slightly differs) of that supervision arrangement, bearing in mind that these may change over time. On a review of the academic literature on supervision it is also clear that the purposes and tasks of supervision vary across professions. Discussion on the purposes and tasks of supervision for therapists contrasts considerably with discussions on supervision for trainee psychiatrists, with one difference simply being more literature available on supervision for therapy and therapists. In fact, most discussion on supervision is to be found in the therapy literature.

Carroll (1996) identifies seven generic tasks of supervision, which are: to create a learning relationship, to teach, to consult, to counsel, to monitor professional and ethical issues, to evaluate, and to monitor the administrative aspect of practice. Kadushin (1976) produces a simpler model, preferring the term 'functions' which are split three ways into educational, supportive and managerial. Proctor (1988) similarly describes the 'formative, restorative and normative' functions, roughly equating with Kadushin's model. Different models of supervision place different emphases on these functions.

For psychiatrists the overarching purpose of supervision is concerned with training and education. Supervision enables training programmes to be evaluated and trainees to be assessed, as well as given career guidance. It may also deal with day-to-day issues arising directly from patient care given that a trainee's supervisor is usually the consultant with whom they work, with the emphasis on furthering their learning. For trainee psychiatrists the supervisor is in fact often referred to as their 'educational supervisor'. Furthermore, when a psychiatrist has completed their training and is eligible to apply for consultant posts, it is no longer a requirement for them to receive supervision and many (if not most) consultants do not engage in any formal supervision process after completion of training.

Supervision for doctors then, is predominantly concerned with training and its educative function. However, unfortunately, when not associated with career and training needs, it is often associated with under-performing doctors who have perhaps been reported to regulatory bodies with the result that supervision is imposed as a condition of being allowed to continue practising and to reassure the public that proper safeguards are put in place. Thus, supervision, in the minds of doctors, may also come to be associated with monitoring of performance and a form of surveillance. This is an example of supervision being more organisation-centred than supervisee-centred, with emphasis on patient protection rather than doctor support.

Arguably, a further example of organisation-centred supervision is a preoccupation with the managerial functions of supervision (as distinct from clinical supervision), more so as the health care culture has become dominated by issues of accountability, standards, clinical governance and performance management. The productivity and efficiency of staff (and therefore of the organisation) are key concerns for managers. Given that supervision is not mandatory, ensuring that managerial agendas are met may have contributed to the development of separate and more clearly delineated processes such as 'individual performance review' (IPR), which is concerned with quality assurance and part of clinical governance. 'Case-load supervision' which can take on managerial functions may also take precedence over 'clinical supervision', the latter usually considered to be the opportunity for the development of reflective practice and attending to learning needs. This seems to indicate that managerial concerns take precedence over the education and support needs of staff.

The supportive aspect of supervision may be demonstrated in several ways. In my experience it is shown by a concern for how I experience my work and conveys the message that how I feel towards what I do is important in its own right, and not simply or solely because it is linked to my effectiveness and productivity. Supervision enables me to talk freely about my mental health and well-being by providing a space in which I do not feel defensive or afraid of the consequences of being honest, where that honesty might reveal health issues. Likewise I can take the time I need to explore what I perceive my needs to be in order to minimise or cope with stress, without feeling awkward or embarrassed talking about my needs. Further examples of how my person-centred supervisor supports me are discussed in the next section. Suffice it to say here, though, that one of the key aspects of feeling supported is feeling valued. I wonder how many mental health professionals come away from a supervision session with an enhanced sense of their own value as both a person and professional?

Common characteristics of supervision

'... a working alliance between a supervisor and a worker or workers in which the worker can reflect on herself in her situation by giving an account of her work and receiving feedback and where appropriate guidance and appraisal. The object of this alliance is to maximise the competence of the worker in providing a helping service.' (Inskipp and Proctor, 1988)

This description of supervision would not seem out of place in mental health settings, for any type of professional. It also illustrates several common characteristics of supervision that I wish to highlight, partly because they contrast with person-centred approaches to supervision.

First, the idea of giving an account of one's work in order to receive feedback puts the supervisor in the position of judge with supervision being a process of external evaluation. The danger of this is that it may lead to a defensive supervisee who significantly edits accounts of his or her work to avoid negative judgements. In addition, the supervisee learns not to trust his or her own judgements and evaluations and relies on an external authority. In person-centred terms he or she is not being encouraged to develop an internal 'locus of evaluation' (the ability to rely on one's own judgements and trust one's own experience and opinions).

Second, and related to this, is the notion of the supervisor being the expert and authority with the inevitable power imbalance this creates in the relationship. The expertise of the supervisor is illustrated by a description of the supervisory process as one that creates 'an inevitable tension as the supervisor gradually lights up the bits that, as they dawn, the PMH [psychiatric mental health] nurse would rather push back into the shadows again' (Wilkin, 2003, p. 545). In other words, in Wilkin's view the supervisor is the one who knows and it is their job to see things the supervisee doesn't, to offer interpretations and to challenge.

A third characteristic suggested by Inskipp and Proctor is one I have already hinted at. It is the idea of using supervision to increase the productivity of the worker and the service they work for.

'Competencies' is a frequently used term in today's NHS when describing the skills, knowledge and activities of mental health professionals. Supervision may be used to enhance those competencies by focusing on the numerous technical aspects, tasks and roles of being a mental health professional. Many of these competencies are of a *doing* nature. This leads me to note a fourth characteristic which is that supervision may concentrate upon problem solving, 'action learning' and on what one *does* as a mental health professional rather than on who one *is*.

Supervision from a person-centred perspective

A person-centred theory of supervision

Rogers does not develop a theory of supervision. In fact, according to Hitchings (2004) he says little about the specific practice of supervision, although he does discuss reflective practice and learning. The development of a person-centred theory of supervision has recently been most fully undertaken by Tudor and Worrall (2004b) and it is based on Rogers' theory of therapy and personality change.

In this person-centred model Tudor and Worrall analyse in the context of supervision the six conditions for constructive personality change Rogers identifies as necessary and sufficient. They accept the 'primacy and centrality of the organism's tendency to actualise' (p. 17), and are interested in which conditions are relevant to supervision and to enhancing the supervisee's tendency to actualise. Rogers' description of the process of therapy (1967) is the template to describe the process of supervision with its various outcomes. (Outcomes here do not describe end-points; rather, they are 'convenient markers of process, particular pauses, points or plateaux to which we give a name and by which we can distinguish the present from the past' (Tudor and Worrall, 2004b, p. 23).) However, for these authors the most important factor in supervision is being empathically understood and unconditionally accepted.

Some characteristics of person-centred supervision

In this section I describe some of the characteristics of a person-centred approach to supervision. I am particularly interested in how values, as well as theory, inform the supervision process and the relationship between supervisor and supervisee. Because some of these characteristics are very general, they can be applied across many professional disciplines in which the supervisee is in a helping relationship. The relevance of what follows is certainly not limited to the supervision of therapists.

Just as attention to the quality of the relationship with patients and clients is the foundation of the person-centred approach, so it is with the supervisory relationship. It may be obvious to highlight the significance of the relationship, yet the distinctiveness of a person-centred approach to relationship with patients and clients is mirrored by the distinctiveness of the supervisory relationship.

Another assumption that can be made about person-centred supervision is its facilitation of the development of the supervisee, but not only professional development in the form of developing competencies and skills. The person-centred approach emphasises the development of the *person* of the helper. The person-centred approach to relationship aims to facilitate the development of the person in which increasing self-awareness will be an outcome. There are many dimensions to self-awareness and in the next section I will describe some of the ways in which person-centred supervision has enhanced my self-awareness. One conclusion to draw from the emphasis on the development of the person in the person-centred approach is that, 'distinctions between professional development and personal growth are at best arbitrary and meaningless' (Worrall, 2001, p. 207).

I have highlighted the crucial need for mental health professionals to feel supported and also how supervision within the NHS often concentrates on the educational and managerial functions of supervision, at the expense of the supportive function. The supportive nature of person-centred supervision is one of its key characteristics in my view, not least because of the freedom and space for the supervisee to discuss their experience in a facilitative environment, but also because of the unconditionally accepting and empathic attitudes the supervisor experiences and communicates. This has been my experience, as I will now go on to describe, along with the many other aspects of my experience of person-centred supervision.

My experience and use of person-centred supervision

In this final section I draw upon some of my experiences of supervision with a person-centred therapist and supervisor who also has an understanding of the workings of NHS mental health services, but who does not work in the same NHS Trust nor has any managerial responsibilities for my work. For me it is important that he understands something of the practicalities, politics and philosophies within my world of work, as well as having no line-management responsibility that may create conflicts of interest. I can be confident that my agenda is paramount and that supervision is not influenced by organisational issues, save those I choose to talk about. I also regard his willingness to let me decide the agenda for our sessions as a mark of his trust in me to know what is important for me to bring and to decide what is most pressing to talk about and explore. I value his non-directive attitude and the way in which supervision takes the form of what Merry calls 'collaborative inquiry' (2002, p. 173) that 'acknowledges that both people involved are self-directed and both can contribute equally to the process' (p. 174). I should probably point out that I also have a supervision arrangement with the consultant with whom I work, who is also my line-manager. This is an expectation according to my particular career grade. This means that in general I am free to use my sessions with my person-centred supervisor exclusively, and in particular, for both receiving support and for developing self-awareness and reflective capacities.

The more we honour and attend to the relationship in our work as mental health professionals, the more self-awareness is important. However, to neglect the development of reflective capacities and the importance of being accurately aware of what is going on for us, is, in my view, to neglect a vital part of being a competent and safe mental health professional, whether we work primarily in a therapeutic way or not. It is important though, to qualify further what I mean by self-awareness and to think about what, specifically, it is important to be aware of. I have already mentioned being aware of our general health, well-being and recognition of our wounds and vulnerabilities. To this should be added an awareness of how our health and well-being impact on our work, relationships with colleagues and patients, and vice versa – how work affects our health and well-being. With this I would include an awareness of our personality traits and general emotional patterns. I may use supervision to explore (and off-load) certain emotions when they threaten to overwhelm me, such as anger, despair or feelings of powerlessness. Likewise, I may notice in supervision when I have become rather emotionally detached or when I retreat into intellectualisation and the comfort of apparently objective certainties.

I also use supervision to explore what I believe about human nature, the assumptions I make about the mind and the brain and what I believe about the nature of mental disturbance and what influences its development. I agree with Merry who believes that if it is our task to enter into the subjective world of others, we also need to question what assumptions we make about the nature of human beings (2002). Regarding person-centred assumptions, I may use supervision to question whether and how much I believe in the human organism's tendency to actualise and what influences my trust or lack of trust in this tendency. I am also interested in what has informed my beliefs about human beings, particularly my own experiences, upbringing and cultural beliefs. Supervision may also provide me with a space to become more aware of some of the big questions such as the nature of freedom, self-determination, responsibility and power, and how my beliefs about these impact on my work.

As well as using supervision to open up philosophical and theoretical issues and enable greater awareness of my core values, supervision also facilitates awareness of my attitudes and feelings towards patients. In particular, I explore the conditions of congruence, unconditional positive regard and empathy and I am able to discover what may block or hinder their development. I become aware of what 'conditions of worth' I impose on patients (the conditions patients have to meet to be accepted and valued – discussed in Chapter 2), what prejudices I carry that make me judgemental and the sorts of situations, problems and patient characteristics in which my empathic sensitivities seem to disappear. I am also aware of how the NHS mental health culture influences, or rather, hinders the development of my congruence, unconditional positive regard and empathic understanding, and in supervision I am able to be more understanding towards myself when I regularly fail to embody the attitudes and values I aspire to.

Another area of self-awareness concerns those inner conflicts and tensions I experience through being a psychiatrist who tries to practise the person-centred approach. These include, for example, issues around my use of the medical model (of assessment, diagnosis and treatment), the non-directive attitude, issues concerning autonomy, responsibility, power and expertise, explaining versus understanding, and the way I approach relationships with patients and colleagues. In this respect it has been important to have a supervisor who is more easily able to empathise with some of the tensions and dilemmas I regularly face trying to be person-centred in the current mental health culture.

My supervisor's ability to understand empathically many of the particular struggles in my work is matched by my experience of his unconditional positive regard and congruence. It is because he offers me a space in which I do not feel judged (either in an evaluative sense or in the sense of communicating critical attitudes) that I am able to explore issues and feelings without fear. This minimises the risk of my defensively distorting or denying my experience. I am more likely to develop congruence, i.e. become more accurately aware of my inner experiencing. His acceptance (unconditional positive regard) of me also facilitates my increasing self-acceptance. This is important because, as Rogers says, '... if I can form a helping relationship to myself – if I can be sensitively aware of and acceptant toward my own feelings – then the likelihood is great that I can form a helping relationship toward another' (1967, p. 51).

In all these ways I feel supported by my supervisor. Not only is what I *do* recognised and validated; *I* am recognised and validated – as both a person and a professional. I would like to end this section by using an analogy I have used elsewhere to describe the supportive function of my supervisor. I describe working in the NHS as a mental health professional as akin to attempting twelve rounds in a boxing ring. I describe my supervisor as my ' "second", the person who waits in the corner of the ring, provides me with refreshment, dries me down with a towel, offers me a bucket to spit in, and gives me vital words of support and encouragement' (Freeth, 2004, p. 262).

Conclusion

It may seem that all this is a lot to ask of supervision and indeed, I think it is. This is why it is important to regard supervision as only one, albeit a potentially invaluable, form of support. I think mental health professionals need to consider where else they may find support. This may include relationships with colleagues, formal and informal networks and seeking out like-minded people who share similar values and attitudes and who speak the same language. Supervision is also only one forum in which we can attend to our personal development and increasing self-awareness. Again, if we take personal development seriously then I think it becomes necessary to seek opportunities that may facilitate its development such as peer groups, workshops and personal learning groups. Reading literature and travel are rich methods of, for example, enhancing empathic understanding by enlarging our outlook and understanding of human nature and the world. In the end, developing reflective capacities and self-awareness will depend upon our attitude to ourselves and to our lives.

We need to be proactive in looking after ourselves, and it may be that working in mental health environments is not consistent with our well-being. If this is the case then it is probably necessary to remove ourselves from these damaging environments. I believe it is also a professional and ethical obligation to ensure that we take care of ourselves in order that we may care more effectively for others. If we cannot attend to our own needs, attending to those of others is likely to be greatly diminished.

Finally, we must never forget the good stories and the positive moments. We must nurture and remember those instances in our work when we feel good about who we are and what we do and where we get the sense that we do make a positive difference.

References

Adshead G (2005) Healing ourselves: ethical issues in the care of sick doctors. *Advances in Psychiatric Treatment,* **11**: 330–337.

Barker P, Manos E, Novak V and Reynolds B (1998) The wounded healer and the myth of mental well-being: ethical issues concerning the mental health status of psychiatric nurses. In P Barker and B Davidson (eds) *Psychiatric Nursing. Ethical Strife.* Arnold, London.

Carroll M (1996) *Counselling Supervision: Theory, Skills and Practice.* Cassell, London.

Freeth R (1996) How much do we matter? *The Doctors' Post,* 5th July, p. 8.

Freeth R (2004) A Psychiatrist's Experience of Person-Centred Supervision. In K Tudor and M Worrall (eds) *Freedom to Practise. Person-centred approaches to supervision.* PCCS Books, Ross-on-Wye, pp. 247–266.

Gilbert J (2004) Supporting Staff. In T Ryan and J Pritchard (eds) *Good Practice in Adult Mental Health.* Jessica Kingsley Publishers, London, pp. 164–182.

Ghodse H (2000) Doctors and their health. Who heals the healers? In H Ghodse, S Mann and P Johnson (eds) *Doctors and their health.* Reed Health Care Limited, Sutton, Surrey, pp. 10–14.

Hitchings P (2004) On Supervision across Theoretical Orientations. In K Tudor and M Worrall (eds) *Freedom to Practise. Person-centred approaches to supervision.* PCCS Books, Ross-on-Wye, pp. 203–224.

Inskipp F and Proctor B (1988) *Skills for Supervising and Being Supervised* (cassette). Cascade Publications, Middlesex.

Kadushin A (1976) *Supervision in Social Work.* Columbia University Press, New York.

Merry T (2002) *Learning and Being in Person-Centred Counselling* (2nd edition). PCCS Books, Ross-on-Wye.

Proctor B (1988) Supervision: A co-operative exercise in accountability. In M Marken and M Payne (eds) *Enabling and Ensuring.* Leicester National Youth Bureau/Council for Education and Training in Youth and Community Work, Leicester.

Redfield Jamison K (1995) *An Unquiet Mind. A Memoir of Moods and Madness.* Picador, London.

Rippere V and Williams R (eds) (1985) *Wounded Healers. Mental Health Workers' Experiences of Depression.* Wiley, Chichester.

Roberts G (2000) Burnout and how to survive it. In H Ghodse, S Mann and P Johnson (eds) *Doctors and their health.* Reed Health Care Limited, Sutton, Surrey, pp. 36–43.

Rogers C (1967) *On Becoming a Person. A Therapist's View of Psychotherapy.* Constable, London.

Tudor K and Worrall M (2004a) Person-Centred Perspectives on Supervision. In K Tudor and M Worrall (eds) *Freedom to Practise. Person-centred approaches to supervision.* PCCS Books, Ross-on-Wye, pp. 43–63.

Tudor K and Worrall M (2004b) Person-Centred Philosophy and Theory in the Practice of Supervision. In K Tudor and M Worrall (eds) *Freedom to Practise. Person-centred approaches to supervision.* PCCS Books, Ross-on-Wye, pp. 11–30.

Walsh B and Walsh S (2001) Is mental health work psychologically hazardous for staff? A critical review of the literature. *Journal of Mental Health,* **10(2):** 121–129.

Wilkin P (2003) Clinical Supervision. In P Barker (ed) *Psychiatric and Mental Health Nursing. The craft of caring.* Arnold, London, pp. 543–551.

Worrall M (2001) Supervision and Empathic Understanding. In S Haugh and T Merry (eds) *Rogers' Therapeutic Conditions: Evolution, Theory and Practice, Volume 2. Empathy.* PCCS Books, Ross-on-Wye, pp. 206–217.

ƐƮƮ

Epilogue

'We must become the change we want to see in the world.'
(Mohandas Gandhi, 1869–1948)

Throughout the process of writing this book I have noticed two things in particular. The first is how much more politically aware I have become; specifically, of how the current political climate dictates the way mental health services are organised and mental health care practised. The second is the increasingly difficult and painful question I regularly ask myself concerning whether I can continue to try to be person-centred as a psychiatrist in such a climate.

It distresses me to need to consider how to maintain my basic humanity within a system that has become, amongst other things, mechanistic, protocol-driven, depersonalised, and a fertile breeding ground for cynicism. It distresses me to witness the corrosive effects of a system of care that devalues persons and the uniqueness of individuals, in the quest for material efficiency, economic supremacy and a striving for the competitive edge. I am often left wondering whether or how much it is possible to cultivate the spirit and values of the person-centred approach in mental health settings that are dominated by logical positivism, reductionism and the medical model, and where power and expertise are assumed to reside mainly in mental health professionals.

In this book I have tried to hold a vision for the practice of the person-centred approach in mental health settings, whilst drawing attention to major philosophical and theoretical differences between this approach and much of psychiatric practice. This book's purpose has primarily been educational, but I also realise I have been trying to articulate my vision of a service that is not dominated by the processes of pathologisation and medicalisation, and in which staff are valued rather than treated as commodities. I believe the person-centred approach can fulfil much of this vision.

I realise these are strong words, but it is with some urgency that, in my opinion, wider social and political change is needed to create a society in which human beings can become more fully human, can be creative, celebrate life, learn to love and to receive love, entertain hope and trust, and genuinely and effectively care for those experiencing mental distress and disturbance. In short, I believe a new paradigm is needed and that the person-centred approach has the potential to contribute to a new paradigm of values and care that may lead to a more healthy society.

Index